Global change and health

Understanding Public Health

Series editors: Nick Black and Rosalind Raine, London School of Hygiene & Tropical Medicine

Throughout the world, recognition of the importance of public health to sustainable, safe and healthy societies is growing. The achievements of public health in nineteenth-century Europe were for much of the twentieth century overshadowed by advances in personal care, in particular in hospital care. Now, with the dawning of a new century, there is increasing understanding of the inevitable limits of individual health care and of the need to complement such services with effective public health strategies. Major improvements in people's health will come from controlling communicable diseases, eradicating environmental hazards, improving people's diets and enhancing the availability and quality of effective health care. To achieve this, every country needs a cadre of knowledgeable public health practitioners with social, political and organizational skills to lead and bring about changes at international, national and local levels.

This is one of a series of 20 books that provides a foundation for those wishing to join in and contribute to the twenty-first-century regeneration of public health, helping to put the concerns and perspectives of public health at the heart of policy-making and service provision. While each book stands alone, together they provide a comprehensive account of the three main aims of public health: protecting the public from environmental hazards, improving the health of the public and ensuring high quality health services are available to all. Some of the books focus on methods, others on key topics. They have been written by staff at the London School of Hygiene & Tropical Medicine with considerable experience of teaching public health to students from low, middle and high income countries. Much of the material has been developed and tested with postgraduate students both in face-to-face teaching and through distance learning.

The books are designed for self-directed learning. Each chapter has explicit learning objectives, key terms are highlighted and the text contains many activities to enable the reader to test their own understanding of the ideas and material covered. Written in a clear and accessible style, the series will be essential reading for students taking postgraduate courses in public health and will also be of interest to public health practitioners and policy-makers.

Titles in the series

Analytical models for decision making: Colin Sanderson and Reinhold Gruen
Controlling communicable disease: Norman Noah
Economic analysis for management and policy: Stephen Jan, Lilani Kumaranayake,
    Jenny Roberts, Kara Hanson and Kate Archibald
Economic evaluation: Julia Fox-Rushby and John Cairns (eds)
Environmental epidemiology: Paul Wilkinson (ed)
Environment, health and sustainable development: Megan Landon
Environmental health policy: David Ball
Financial management in health services: Reinhold Gruen and Anne Howarth
Global change and health: Kelley Lee and Jeff Collin (eds)
Health care evaluation: Sarah Smith, Don Sinclair, Rosalind Raine and Barnaby Reeves
Health promotion practice: Maggie Davies, Wendy Macdowall and Chris Bonell (eds)
Health promotion theory: Maggie Davies and Wendy Macdowall (eds)
Introduction to epidemiology: Lucianne Bailey, Katerina Vardulaki, Julia Langham and
    Daniel Chandramohan
Introduction to health economics: David Wonderling, Reinhold Gruen and Nick Black
Issues in public health: Joceline Pomerleau and Martin McKee (eds)
Making health policy: Kent Buse, Nicholas Mays and Gill Walt
Managing health services: Nick Goodwin, Reinhold Gruen and Valerie Iles
Medical anthropology: Robert Pool and Wenzel Geissler
Principles of social research: Judith Green and John Browne (eds)
Understanding health services: Nick Black and Reinhold Gruen

Global change and health

Edited by Kelley Lee and Jeff Collin

Open University Press

Open University Press
McGraw-Hill Education
McGraw-Hill House
Shoppenhangers Road
Maidenhead
Berkshire
England
SL6 2QL

email: enquiries@openup.co.uk
world wide web: www.openup.co.uk

and Two Penn Plaza, New York, NY 10121-2289, USA

First published 2005

A catalogue record of this book is available from the British Library

ISBN-10: 0 335 21848 2 (pb)
ISBN-13: 978 0 335 21848 6 (pb)

Library of Congress Cataloging-in-Publication Data
CIP data applied for

Typeset by RefineCatch Limited, Bungay, Suffolk
Printed in Poland EU by OZGraf S.A.
www.polskabook.pl

Contents

Acknowledgements

Open University Press and the London School of Hygiene and Tropical Medicine have made every effort to obtain permission from copyright holders to reproduce material in this book and to acknowledge these sources correctly. Any omissions brought to our attention will be remedied in future editions.

We would like to express our grateful thanks to the following copyright holders for granting permission to reproduce material in this book.

p. 10   American Automobile Manufacturers Association, *World Motor Vehicle Data*,
p. 44   Bellamy C, *The State of the World's Children 2002*, UNICEF.
p. 22   National Center for Health Statistics. *Health*, United States, 2004. With Chartbook on Trends in the Health of Americans. Hyattsville, Maryland: 2004
p. 150   Commission on Human Security, *Human Security Now*, 2003.
p. 76   Cornia GA, Globalization and health: results and options, *Bulletin of the World Health Organization*, 2001, 79(9):834–841.
p.14   Dahlgren G and Whitehead M (1991), *Policies and Strategies to Promote Social Equity in Health*. Stockholm, Institute of Futures Studies.
p. 85   Reprinted by permission of Sage Publications Ltd from Dicken P, *Global shift 3rd edition*, Copyright (© Peter Dicken, 1998).
p. 75   *Globalization, Growth and poverty: Building and inclusive world economy* by Dollar, David . Copyright 2001 by WORLD BANK. Reproduced with permission of WORLD BANK in the format Textbook via Copyright Clearance Center.
pp. 74, 75 *Policy Research Working Papers* by Dollar, David. Copyright 2001 by WORLD BANK. Reproduced with permission of WORLD BANK in the format Textbook via Copyright Clearance Center
p. 157   Reprinted by permission of *FOREIGN AFFAIRS*, (81; 6; November/December 2002). Copyright (2002) by the Council on Foreign Relations, Inc.
pp. 77–81 Feachem R, 'Globalisation is good for your health, mostly,' *BMJ*, 2001, 323:504–506, with permission from the BMJ Publishing Group.
p. 149   Fidler D, Public Health and National security in the Global Age: Infectious Diseases, Bioterrorism and Realpolitik, *George Washington International Law Review*, 2003, 35(4):787–856.
pp. 166, 175 Fidler D. SARS, *Governance, and the Globalization of Disease*, 2004, Palgrave Macmillan, reproduced with permission of Palgrave Macmillan'.
p. 155   Heinecken L, Living in Terror: The looming security threat to Southern Africa, *African Security Review*, 2001, 10(4), Institute of Security Studies.
p. 24   Fig 2.8 Predicted trends in BMI for England, Mauritius and Brazil (1960–2030), International Obesity Task Force (IOTF) [no date].
p. 101   Light, 'Counterveiling framework for professions in transition', in T Johnson, G Larkin and M Saks, *Health professions and the state in Europe*, p37, Routledge, 1995.
p. 113   Lopez A et al (eds), 'A descriptive model of the cigarette epidemic in developed countries,' *Tobacco Control*, 1994, 3:242–249, reproduced with permission from the BMJ Publishing Group.
p. 23   Martorell, R. 2001. Obesity. In Health and Nutrition: Emerging and

	Reemerging Issues in Developing Countries, ed. Rafael Flores and Stuart Sillespie. *2020 Vision Focus 5*. Washington DC: International Food Research Institute. Reproduced with permission from
p. 106	McKeown T, *The Modern Rise of Population*, Edward Arnold, 1976, copyright. Reproduced by permission of Edward Arnold.
p. 142	McMichael A et al, *Human health and climate change in Oceania: a risk assessment 2002*, copyright Commonwealth of Australia reproduced by permission.
p. 139	McMichael AJ, *Planetary overload: global environmental change and the health of the human species*, 1993, Cambridge University Press.
p. 149	National Intelligence Council, 'National Intelligence Estimate: The global infectious disease threat and its implications for the US,' 2000, *Environmental Change and Security Project Report*, 6, (Summer 2000), Central Intelligence Agency.
pp. 141–144	J Patz, Global Warning, BMJ, 2004, 328:1269–1270, with permission from the BMJ Publishing Group.
p. 64	Scholte JA, *What is 'global' about globalization?*, 2000, Palgrave Macmillan, reproduced with permission of Palgrave Macmillan.
p. 201	Seckinelgin H, 'Time to stop and think: HIV/AIDS, global civil society, and people's politics,' *Global Civil Society*, 2002, Oxford University Press.
p. 113	Shafey O, Dolwick S, Guindon GE (eds). Tobacco Control Country Profiles 2003, *American Cancer Society*, Atlanta, GA, 2003.
p. 199	Thomas A, 'Non-governmental organisations and the limits to empowerment' in *Development Policy and Public Action*, T Hewitt, M Wuyats and M Mackintosh (eds), 1993. By permission of Oxford University Press.
pp. 17, 18	UNESCO, Study on International flows of cultural goods between 1980–98, reproduced by permission of UNESCO.
pp. 17, 18	UNESCO, World Trade of Cultural goods (in millions of dollars), 1980–98, reproduced by permission of UNESCO. http://portal.unesco.org/culture/en/ev.php-URL_ID=18669&URL_DO=DO_TOPIC&URL_SECTION=201.html
p. 115	UNESCO, Cutural, trade and globalisation, questions & Answers, reproduced by permission of UNESCO. http://portal.unesco.org/culture/en/ev.php-URL_ID=18669&URL_DO=DO_TOPIC&URL_SECTION=201.html
p. 87	World Health Organization, *Building Block for tobacco control: A handbook*, 2004, reproduced with permission from World Health Organization.
p. 92	World Trade Organization, *Understanding the WTO*, 2003, reproduced with permission from World Trade Organization.

Data sources only:

p. 68	Fortune 2000.
p. 96	IMS Health Top Companies, July 2004.
p. 11	International Telecommunication Union, 2001.

Overview of the book

The subject of *global health* is a relatively new but rapidly expanding one as scholars and public health practitioners recognize the important challenges that global changes are posing for human health. The starting point for this book is the identification of a broad shift from *international* to *global* health. This shift can be said to be occurring where the determinants of health circumvent, undermine or are oblivious to the territorial boundaries of states and, therefore, effectively addressing health outcomes exceeds the capacity of individual countries acting alone through domestic institutions. The issue areas covered in this book are selected to provide the reader with an introductory understanding of the multiple ways in which health is affected by global change.

Why study global change and health?

The subject of globalization remains under considerable debate, and there are diverse and often strikingly divergent views expressed. Bound up in these views are varying personal experiences of globalization, as well as conflicting opinions on how these processes should be played out. From a health perspective, the debate is further clouded by the relative scarcity of evidence available to date concerning the causal connections between global changes taking place and their health implications. In some cases, these connections may be quite direct; in other cases, there can be intervening variables which makes determining causality much more complex. Thus, while global health is attracting considerable attention, the existing literature remains disparate and uneven in its empirical underpinnings.

As such, this book cannot be comprehensive and treatment of each issue area must inevitably be limited. Nonetheless, the book offers clarification of the parameters of global health as an emerging field. It explores areas where there is emerging evidence that a shift is taking place. By the end of this book, you will be encouraged to think differently about health – what it means and how it is achieved – within the context of the changing world around us.

Structure of the book

The book begins with an introduction to global health as a subject area. It sets out a conceptual framework for understanding different types of global change taking place, the key drivers of globalization, and the main features of the shift from international to global health. The remainder of the book combines broad overviews addressing how global change is impacting on the social, economic, environmental and political spheres with chapters focused on key specific issues. Some such chapters encourage you to think anew about familiar health issues from a global perspective (e.g. food policy, infectious disease, pharmaceuticals, tobacco control), while others which show how other policy areas and agendas are impacting on health (e.g. gender, trade, security). The book concludes with three chapters on the challenges for developing global health governance – assessing the kinds of institutions and actions that are needed to meet the challenges facing us all. Each chapter includes:

- an overview
- learning objectives
- a list of key terms
- a range of activities
- feedback on those activites (where appropriate)
- a summary

Acknowledgements

The editors acknowledge the generosity of the WHO in permitting use of material developed for its training course on 'Public Health Implications of the WTO Multilateral Trade Agreements' and thank Nadja Doyle, Melanie Batty and Louise Evans for their efficient and patient support and Deirdre Byrne (series manager) for help and advice.

Introduction to global health

Overview

This chapter provides an introduction to the emerging field of global health. It begins by defining the often used, yet highly debated, term globalization. This is accompanied by a conceptual framework for understanding its distinct features. A discussion of why globalization is happening – the key technological, economic and political drivers – then follows. Finally, the chapter concludes with a discussion of the emerging shift from international to global health arising as a result of globalization.

Learning objectives

After working through this chapter, you will be able to:

- **define the concepts of global change and globalization, and the key debates surrounding them**
- **describe a conceptual framework for understanding the linkages between globalization and health**
- **identify the various drivers and forms of global change (e.g. environmental, economic)**

Key terms

Dimensions of global change The three types of changes – spatial, temporal and cognitive – taking place that characterize globalization.

Global health A health issue where the determinants circumvent, undermine or are oblivious to the territorial boundaries of states and, thus, beyond the capacity of individual countries to address through domestic institutions.

Globalization A set of global processes that are changing the nature of human interaction across a wide range of social spheres including the economic, political, cultural and environmental.

What does globalization mean?

It is easy to become overwhelmed by the subject of globalization given widespread interest among policy makers, the business community, academia, mass media and the general public. The term has generated an ever growing literature which threatens to swamp even the most enthusiastic reader. Nor is this literature cohesive in content or perspective. Newcomers to the field must immediately recognize that the term 'globalization' is highly contested and still under debate. There are four main points of debate within the vast globalization literature:

• Is globalization actually happening or not? Is what is happening actually new?
• What are the reasons behind what is happening? What are the causes or drivers?
• What is the timeframe for what is happening? Is it a recent phenomenon or does it have historical roots?
• What impacts is globalization having? Are these impacts positive or negative, good or bad?

Certainly a lot of people are talking about globalization, many of whom have strong and often opposed views about the subject. The task of this chapter, therefore, is not simply to present you with the 'facts'. Many of these so-called 'facts' are contested depending on who you are, what values you hold, how rich you happen to be and so on. We cannot provide you with an easy resolution of these conflicting views. What you can be is informed about what kinds of debates are taking place and the different perspectives being put forth on various issues. It will then be up to you to think about your own lives, weigh up the evidence, sort through different value systems, and then decide how you stand on these issues.

We can begin by attempting to define globalization more clearly. There are many different definitions of globalization available – some of which are partly right, some of which are quite wrong as when the term is used to re-label previously existing phenomenon.

Here are a few examples of quite diverse definitions of globalization:

• '. . . a global shopping mall in which ideas and products are available every-where at the same time'. Kanter (1995)
• 'what we in the Third World have for several centuries called colonization'. Khor (1995)

and

• 'a stretching of social, political and economic activities across frontiers such that events, decisions and activities in one region of the world can come to have significance for individuals and communities in distant regions of the globe'. Held et al. (1999)

Kanter (1995) sees globalization as a rather positive thing in terms of the consumer society and the benefit to shoppers of more things to buy. Khor (1995), from the non-governmental organization (NGO) Third World Network, is far more critical, seeing globalization as an extension of colonization of the developing world. Held et al. (1999) see globalization as a more complex set of processes, focusing on how events, decisions and activities in one part of the world can have consequences in other parts of the world. This is often referred to as a greater interdependence or interrelatedness of the world.

There are some sceptics who question whether globalization is actually happening at all. Hirst and Thompson (1995) argue that we are not seeing anything different, and claims are much exaggerated. They believe we have always had different societies trading with one another, indeed at times in the past more so than today. Glyn and Sutcliffe (1992) take a similar line, arguing that it is not much different from the international economy we had one hundred or so years ago. They argue that the world was more integrated economically during the Industrial Revolution.

 Activity 1.1

Select a national newspaper in your country that you have daily access to. For one week scan and clip any stories and articles using the words 'global' or 'globalization'. Make a file of your clippings.

Is globalization defined and if so, how? Make a note of the various definitions of globalization used. Where it is not defined, is a definition implied? If possible identify who holds the definition – government official, corporate executive, NGO worker and so on. What aspect of globalization does each story focus upon (e.g. economic, environmental, social)? Do the articles identify any winners and losers from globalization? Try to decide if each story presents a positive or negative perspective on globalization.

A conceptual framework for understanding globalization and health

This book argues that there is something called 'globalization' happening even if many people cannot seem to agree what it is. The world is changing in distinct ways, and in some cases these changes are having unprecedented impacts on human health. If we put aside the rather tangled mess of definitions found in the existing literature, we can begin by thinking about what is distinct. How we might describe how the world is changing. What are we experiencing as changing around us?

One framework for understanding globalization is to focus on three dimensions of global change: spatial, temporal and cognitive. First, globalization is leading to changes to human societies along the *spatial dimension*. Globalization is creating changes to how we perceive and experience physical or territorial space. This is perhaps the easiest aspect of globalization for us to grasp. The physical world, of course, is the same size as it has always been. But what is different is how we, as human beings, interact with that space. How we move across territorial space, how we define and use space, and how we interact across physical distances is being changed as a consequence of globalization.

Foremost is the increase in population mobility. Just one generation ago, most people stayed near to where they were born and grew up. Travel was rare, expensive and involved short distances. Since the 1980s, for many people, it has become more affordable to travel over long distances. Travel might be temporary, such as for business, study or due to unexpected displacement. Or travel can be longer term such as when people migrate to settle elsewhere more permanently. Today we are a generation on the move like never before, and trends in increasing population mobility are expected to continue. The following statistics illustrate this:

- It is estimated that almost 175 million people (2.9% of the world's population) were living outside their country of birth in 2000, an increase from 100 million (1.8% of world's population) in 1995, and a more than doubling since 1965 (Stilwell et al., 2004).
- According to the International Labour Organization (ILO), 130 million people worldwide were migrant workers in 2000, an increase from 75 million in 1965.
- The UN High Commissioner for Refugees estimates that the total number of refugees and others of concern to the organization (such as asylum seekers and internally displaced persons) reached 21.8 million in 2000, a substantial increase from 1.4 million in 1961.
- Data from the World Tourism Organization reports that total international arrivals worldwide reached 699 million in 2000 (around 9% of the world's population), representing an annual increase of 7.9%. The number of long haul travellers is expected to reach 377 million by 2020.

As we move around the world, we bring animals (including microbes) and plants, for example, with us either deliberately or unintentionally. This may occur on an individual scale, such as when we harbour a cold or influenza virus, or sometimes something far worse. This was how the outbreak of SARS (severe acute respiratory syndrome) was spread from southern China to 30 other countries. Air travel was a key means by which the outbreak became an epidemic (resulting in a total of 8,422 cases and 916 deaths). The movement of life forms can also occur on a larger scale such as when ships on one side of the world fill up their ballasts with sea water, along with all sorts of marine life, and empty that water at their destination in another part of the world. Indeed, it is believed that this kind of activity has caused so-called 'bio invasions', with native species threatened by the introduction of rival species through human activity. Mass movement of life forms also occurs through flourishing global economic and trade relations. The introduction of cash crops in many parts of the world has displaced many native plant species. Mass production in larger and larger farms has reduced the varieties of certain crops grown, such as corn, wheat and potatoes (see Chapter 4). It is feared that the increased growing of genetically modified organisms (GMO) will accelerate this trend.

The spatial dimension of global change is thus one key aspect of how we can understand globalization. Globalization as spatial charge has been described as:

- 'growth of "supraterritorial" relations between people . . . a far-reaching change in the nature of social space'. Scholte (2000)
- 'processes through which sovereign national states are criss-crossed and undermined by transnational actors'. Beck (1999)

and

- 'intensification of worldwide social relations which link distant localities in such a way that local happenings are shaped by events occurring many miles away and vice versa'. Giddens (1990)

The second dimension of global change is *temporal* – how we perceive and experience time. The link between space and time is a close one. We are able to move about more quickly and across greater distances because of available technologies such as jet airliners and high speed trains. Alternatively, we may not need to cross physical distances anymore to interact with other people because we can use forms of communication, notably the Internet, that are quicker and more accessible than ever before. The experience of an accelerated timeframe can be seen in the following example from medical research. Decoding of genetic sequencing has relied heavily on the computing capacity of prevailing technologies. During the 1970s it took two months to sequence 150 nucleotides, the letters that spell out a gene. It took 1,000 scientists around ten years to decode the first yeast genome. However, due to greater computer processing speeds possible today the same process takes hours instead of years.

However, anyone with an e-mail address will know that globalization may or may not mean a net saving in time. Because of our capacity to interact more readily, we may do so more frequently (and spent more time responding to others). Or we might spend more time travelling because of the availability of cheap flights. In other ways, life seems to have slowed down – dealing with large bureaucracies, negotiating the automated telephone options of a large organization, or finding ourselves stuck on increasingly congested roads. More accurately, therefore, globalization is changing our relationship with time. We are spending our time differently than a generation ago. For a lucky few, enjoying the fruits of globaliza- tion, leisure time may increase relative to working hours. For many, the pressures of life in a 'post-industrial society' can mean juggling an increasing number of commitments. And for others still, the insecurities of work or unemployment means a very different set of pressures. Here are some quotes from writers who describe the temporal dimension of global change:

- 'we have been experiencing, these last two decades, an intense phase of time- space compression that has had a disorienting and disruptive impact'. Harvey (1989)
- 'a growing magnitude or intensity of global flows'. Held and McGrew (2000)

and

- 'global transactions . . . can extend anywhere in the world at the same time and can unite locations anywhere in effectively no time'. Scholte (2000)

The third dimension of change associated with globalization is *cognitive*. This refers to how globalization is changing the what we think about ourselves and the world around us. Some of the main agents of cognitive change are the mass media, advertising agencies, consultancy firms, research and educational institutions, religious groups and political parties. The thought processes being influenced by their activities include cultural values, beliefs, ideologies, policies and knowledge.

Among these, perhaps the most ubiquitous in contemporary societies is the mass media which, in its restructuring and influence, has become global. Until the 1980s, print and broadcast media in most countries were national in scope. There has been trade in books, films, music and television programmes across countries for decades, but broadcasting and publishing industries remained largely domestic in ownership and regulation. Since the 1980s, there has been a technological convergence in modes of communications, and many argue a corresponding convergence in the content of the messages they convey. This has been the result of widespread deregulation and privatization of the telecommunications sector, initially in the US and Europe, and more recently in middle- and low-income countries.

Table 1.1 The 'Big Seven' global media giants (2004)

Company	Revenue	Selected holdings
News Corporation	US$14 billion	20th Century Fox, HarperCollins, Times, STAR TV, BSkyB, New York Post
Viacom	US$12 billion	Paramount, CBS, MTV, Blockbuster Video, Simon & Schuster
Walt Disney	US$25 billion	Disney Films, Miramax, Mammoth Records, ABC, ESPN
AOL Time Warner	US$38 billion	New Line Cinema, HBO, Time Life Books, AOL, Warner Bros, CNN
Sony Corporation	US$58 billion	Columbia Tristar, HBO Asia, Cineplex Odeon, Sony Records
Vivendi Universal	7.3b euro	Universal Studios, Canal+, Polygram, Motown
Bertelsmann	US$13 billion	AOL Europe, Arista Records, Bantam Doubleday, Random House

Source: www.mediachannel.org.

Looking at the mass media in more detail, we see that it is increasingly dominated by a small number of large corporations, many of which are diversifying into different types of print and broadcast media. Table 1.1 lists the seven largest global media conglomerates in 2004.

The substantial revenues of each corporation – which have grown through mergers and acquisitions – are striking. Each company has diverse holdings in a range of print and broadcast media. News Corporation, for example, owns the major television and film production company, 20th Century Fox, as well as the publishing company HarperCollins, the British newspaper *The Times* (along with many others), the US newspaper the *New York Post*, and the satellite broadcasting companies Star TV (Asia) and BSkyB (UK). To these holdings can be added sports teams, retail shops, and even theme parks. Furthermore, the holdings are worldwide. Viacom, Walt Disney and AOL Time Warner are all American-owned companies, but their holdings cannot be described as exclusively American. The global reach of the mass media is reflected in increased international trade of goods with cultural content. From 1980 to 1991 trade tripled from US$67 billion to US$200 billion.

Given the sheer size of these companies and their ability to entertain, inform and sell to us, it is perhaps not surprising that people believe they have the power to influence our thoughts. Here are quotes from writers who describe the cognitive dimension of global change.

- 'the compression of the world and the intensification of consciousness of the world as a whole'. Robertson (1992)
- 'McWorld's homogenization is likely to . . . [lead to] the triumph of commerce and its markets and to give to those who control information, communication, and entertainment ultimate control over human destiny'. Barber (1992)

and

- 'We cannot hope to preserve every culture in the world just as it is. And we cannot want a culture to be preserved if it lacks the internal will and cohesion to do so itself. As with species, cultures spawning, evolving and dying is part of evolution. But what is going on today, thanks to globalization, is turbo-evolution.' Friedman (1999)

To summarize so far, it is important to recognize that globalization is a complex set of processes, drivers and consequences that we need to untangle in order to understand their health impacts. While there tends to be a strong focus on economic globalization – the global economy, capital flows, market restructuring, foreign investment and so on – this is only one face of globalization. Globalization affects many aspects of our lives.

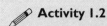 **Activity 1.2**

Refer again to your scrapbook of newspaper clippings on globalization compiled in Activity 1.1. Review the stories again and see if you can identify whether they refer to spatial, temporal or cognitive globalization. Do they discuss economic, political, cultural or environmental change?

The technologies behind globalization

Technology is frequently seen as the key driver of global change. It is the most visible manifestation of the changes around us, enabling us to do the things we associate with globalization. There are two key technological drivers – transportation and information technology. Long-haul flights, bullet trains and super tankers all enable us to move ourselves and our possessions farther and more frequently than ever before. This is because the cost of transport has declined significantly. Table 1.2 describes how transport costs by sea and air have declined during the twentieth century. Sea freight, for example, has dropped from US$95 per tonne to US$29 (in 1990 US$). Larger capacity ships, more efficient engines, fuel costs, and greater market competition all have made it financially cheaper to ship freight by sea. Similarly for air transport, the financial cost per passenger mile has declined about six-fold from US$0.68 to US$0.11 due to technological developments in airplane design and size, economies of scale and keener market competition.

It is important to note, of course, that the associated environmental costs from increased use of transport technologies are not included in these figures. As

Table 1.2 Declining cost of transport (1990 US$)

YEAR	SEA FREIGHT (average ocean freight and port charges per tonne)	AIR TRANSPORT (average revenue per passenger mile)
1920	95	—
1930	60	0.68
1940	63	0.46
1950	34	0.30
1960	27	0.24
1970	27	0.16
1980	24	0.10
1990	29	0.11

Source: UNDP 1999.

explored more fully in Chapter 10, there is growing evidence that the substantial rise in the burning of fossil fuels over the last century has contributed to global warming. More immediately, there is potentially serious damage from oil spills due to increased sea traffic. These 'costs' are created yet largely omitted from any assessment of the price of globalization. Moreover, such costs are borne inequitably. In high-income countries, and in an increasing number of middle-income countries, the advent of the automobile age has added to our personal mobility. There has been a steady and seemingly inexorable increase in the number of motor vehicles on the world's roads. Many of these are private vehicles; many others are trucks carrying freight across countries and even continents. Figure 1.1 illustrates the rising number of motor vehicle registration worldwide between 1945 and 1995. In 1950, there were 70 million cars, trucks and buses worldwide. By 1994, there was about nine times this number (630 million).

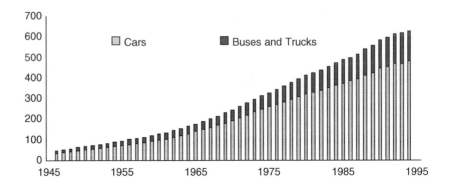

The other key technological driver of globalization is information and communication technologies.

The nineteenth century saw the introduction of telegraphy, followed by radio and telephony by the early twentieth century. Over the next one hundred years, enormous leaps in technology were witnessed – television, undersea cables, satellites, personal computers, facsimile, mobile telephones and the Internet. Figure 1.2 illustrates the steep rise in the use of four technologies – telephone, mobile phone, personal computer and the Internet – during the 1990s.

Again, the main reason for this exponential growth in use has been falling costs. The cost of telephone calls have fallen even more rapidly than transport costs. In 1930, it would have cost US$245 to make a three minute call from London to New York, compared to US$3.00 in 1990 (even allowing for inflation). In 2003, this same telephone call cost US$1.00.

Technological developments have also been a key driver of temporal change. With new technologies, we can do lots of things faster. A good example is the processing speed of computers. The Intel 8086 processor, introduced in 1981, had an average speed of 4.77 megahertz (MHz) and a personal computer with this processor would cost about US$5,000. By the mid-1980s, the Intel 80386 was introduced which was ten times as fast and cost about the same. A decade later computers were five times

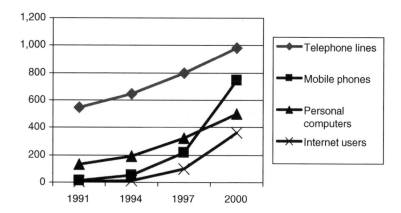

as fast again and had declined in cost (US$3,000). By 2001 processing speeds once again increased ten fold, with costs declining to around US$1,500.

And, of course, processors are not only used in personal computers. They are important for computers used in all sorts of settings, for example, in stock exchanges for worldwide financial trading, by banks to carry out electronic transactions, by airlines to book and coordinate flights and passengers, by retailers to manage stock and other logistics, by the mass media to create and transmit programmes, by telecom companies for sending and receiving information. The increased speed of processors has had widespread uses in society, enabling us to do a whole range of things faster and faster.

✎ Activity 1.3

Make a list of transportation and communication technologies that you use in your work and private life. Can you recall when you began to use these technologies? Now think about how they have changed the way you work and live. Do the technologies allow you to do things differently? Do the technologies allow you to interact with people across time and distance more readily?

Summary

The field of global health is a rapidly emerging one that needs clearer definition and conceptualization. At the heart of global health are changes being brought about by globalization, a highly contested term to describe a greater intensity and extensity of people, other life forms, capital, knowledge and ideas moving across national boundaries. Chapter 2 begins to link globalization with health by considering the realm of social change.

References

American Automobile Manufacturers Association (1993) *World Motor Vehicle Data 1993*. AAMA: Washington DC.

Barber B (1992) 'Jihad vs McWorld'. *Atlantic Monthly*, March; 269: 53–65.

Beck U (1999) *What Is Globalization?* Cambridge: Polity Press.

Friedman T (1999) *The Lexus and the Olive Tree*. New York: HarperCollins.

Giddens A (1990) *The Consequences of Modernity*. Stanford: Stanford University Press.

Glyn A and Sutcliffe R (1992) 'Global but Leaderless? The New Capitalist Order'. *Socialist Register*: 76–95.

Harvey D (1989) *The Condition of Postmodernity*. Oxford: Blackwell.

Held D, McGrew A, Goldblatt D and Perraton J (1999) *Global Transformations, Politics, Economics and Culture*. Stanford: Stanford University Press.

Held D and McGrew A (2000) *The Global Transformations Reader*. London: Polity Press.

Hirst P and Thompson G (1995) 'Globalization and the future of the nation state'. *Economy and Society*, 24(3): 408–42.

Kanter RM (1995) *World Class: Thriving Locally in the Global Economy*. New York: Simon & Schuster.

Khor M (1995) 'Globalization and the Need for Coordinated Southern Policy Response'. *Cooperation South, Special Issue*, New Directions, Special Unit for Technical Cooperation among Developing Countries.

MediaChannel, *Diversity, Democracy And Access: Is Media Concentration A Crisis?* (New York: no date). Available at: http://www.mediachannel.org/ownership/front.shtml#chart.

Robertson R (1992) *Globalization: Social Theory and Global Culture*. London: Sage.

Scholte JA (2000) *Globalization, A Critical Introduction*. London: Macmillan.

Stilwell B, Diallo K, Zurn P, Vujicic M, Adams O and Dal Poz M (2004) 'Migration of health-care workers from developing countries: strategic approaches to its management'. *Bulletin of the World Health Organization*, 82(8): 595–600.

UNDP (1999) *Human Development Report 1999*. New York: United Nations Development Programme.

2 Global social change and health

Overview

Chapter 1 introduced the concept of globalization and how it is contributing to a wide range of changes to human societies around the world. In this chapter, you begin to explore the key question at the heart of this book – what are the linkages between globalization and health? There are a range of changes taking place which can collectively be called globalization. How are these changes, in turn, impacting on our health as individuals and collectively (population health)? In this chapter, you will begin to explore this question in relation to how selected social changes are impacting on health. This concerns how human societies are organized; how individuals live together as families, communities or countries; what cultural beliefs and values are held; and what collective aspirations people have. All of these features hold implications for our health.

Learning objectives

After working through this chapter, you will be able to:

- **understand globalization in relation to the broad determinants of health**
- **describe the increasingly global nature of the consumer society, and the key drivers of these changes**
- **identify selected health issues created by the spread of certain lifestyles and aspirations**
- **recognize the ways in which globalization may be influencing emerging trends in non-communicable disease.**

Key terms

Cultural globalization The blurring of previously accepted boundaries which differentiated states, ethnicities and civil societies such that new spaces of daily life, new sources of cultural meaning, and new forms of social and political agency flow across national borders.

Global society The idea that globalization is leading to people being incorporated into a single world society.

Global village The concept that people are increasingly holding notions of society that combine micro-level (community, district, nationality) and macro-level (world) identities.

Global social change and the broad determinants of health

There is now widespread recognition within the public health community of the broad determinants of health. These determinants range from individual factors, such as genetic makeup, gender and age, and lifestyle choices, to wider social and community influences, to even broader living and working conditions, and general socioeconomic, cultural and environmental conditions.

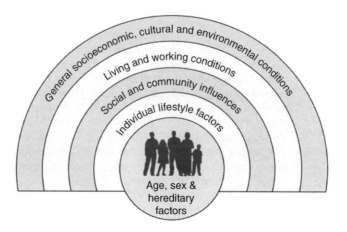

How does globalization fit into this picture? Accumulating evidence about the linkages between globalization and health suggests that the changes taking place are not limited in impact to the outer ring of Figure 2.1. Indeed, the picture is far more complex, with global changes permeating throughout the various layers, for example:

- through population mobility patterns that affect the genetic makeup of populations and hence their susceptibility or protection from certain genetically inherited disorders;
- through the spread of cultural values and beliefs through global marketing and advertising resulting in changing lifestyles and associated health consequences;
- through the spread and adoption of social policies across countries that affect access to health care;
- through global restructuring of the world economy that leads to the employment of workers without appropriate protection under health and safety regulations; and
- through the widening of socioeconomic inequalities within and across many countries, resulting in impoverishment and poorer health for certain population groups.

While it is not possible to explore all of these different layers in this chapter, or within the book as a whole, it is useful to keep this framework in mind when seeking to untangle the complex causal relationships that link globalization and health. To better understand these complex links, the remainder of this chapter considers some key areas of global social change.

Health and the rise of the global consumer

In his definition of globalization, Albrow (1990) writes about the emergence of a 'global society' defined as 'all those processes by which the peoples of the world are incorporated into a single world society, global society.' Debates rage as to the extent to which a global society, as defined, is truly emerging. The evidence is decidedly mixed. Integral to such debates are the impacts of such a trend toward social integration on individual societies, as well as individuals within those societies. Are we experiencing a so-called 'clash of civilizations' (Huntington, 2002) or the emergence of a 'global village'? Whatever is happening, it seems a painful birth at times.

The impacts on human health of global social change are also throwing up mixed messages. There are clear causes for concern in terms of the shift in life-styles, cognitive frameworks, etc leading to adverse consequences. At the same time, there are signs of solidarity across societies in support of progressive ideals such as social justice, environmental sustainability and health as a basic human right.

One of the abiding images at the heart of the globalization concept is that of the 'global village'. This term was coined during the 1960s by the Canadian writer Marshall McLuhan who was reflecting on the experience of living next door to the largest consumer market in the world, the US. He observed that people living in different parts of the world were beginning to share certain values, ideas, beliefs and aspirations. Undoubtedly, McLuhan was under no illusions that many things continued to divide the world. What he described, however, was an emerging sense of community spanning the globe as never before.

The image of a global village is a highly attractive one because it evokes optimism that humanity can share understandings and interests that overcome divisions that have scarred human relations throughout history. Despite its laudable intentions, the idea that current forms of globalization are leading to a global society remains a highly disputed one. Some argue that the global village can more accurately be described as 'global pillage'. Globalization is seen as a colonizing rather than liberating force, enabling a dominant (largely American) culture to dominate the rest of the world. Other writers ask more nuanced questions about the kind of global society that might be emerging. What kinds of values and beliefs underpin the global village? What cultural goods and services bind its citizens together? The extract below, from a UNESCO (2000) publication, explores what is understood by cultural goods and services.

What do we understand by cultural goods and services?

The concepts of 'cultural goods' and 'cultural services', which appear clearly distinct, are sometimes difficult to dissociate. In fact, their respective definitions and meanings are one of the key issues currently being discussed at the international level. The combination of both terms is commonly referred to as 'cultural products', and could be tentatively defined as follows:

- Cultural goods generally refer to those consumer goods that convey ideas, symbols, and ways of life. They inform or entertain, contribute to build collective identity and influence cultural practices. The result of individual or collective creativity – thus copyright-based – cultural goods are reproduced and boosted by industrial processes and worldwide distribution. Books, magazines, multimedia products, software, records, films, videos, audio-visual programmes, crafts and fashion design constitute plural and diversified cultural offerings for citizens at large.
- It is traditionally understood that cultural services are those activities aimed at satisfying cultural interests or needs. Such activities do not represent material goods in themselves: they typically consist of the overall set of measures and supporting facilities for cultural practices that government, private and semi-public institutions or companies make available to the community. Examples of such services include the promotion of performances and cultural events as well as cultural information and preservation (libraries, documentation centres and museums). Cultural services may be offered for free or on a commercial basis.

One of the forces uniting citizens of this so-called global village is a value system based on individual wants and needs. Former British Prime Minister Margaret Thatcher famously once said that 'there is no such thing as society. There are individual men and women, and there are families. And no government can do anything except through people, and people must look to themselves first'. It is this primacy given to the individual, over the collective, that many feel current forms of globalization are defined by.

This is manifest, foremost, in the spread of the consumer society whereby countries around the world have seen a rise in the variety and availability of goods and services produced elsewhere. Through the restructuring of the world economy (see Chapter 7), a growing number of 'global brands' are being produced for consumption by people throughout the world. For some, at least, the global market-place means the same fast food outlets, designer labels, leading brands, popular culture and indeed, entire lifestyles shared with others far away. One of the most famous is the soft drink, Coca-Cola®, whose marketing campaigns recognized early on the potential to attain global status. Perhaps the most famous advertisement of the 1970s showed young people from a variety of ethnic backgrounds holding bottles of Coca-Cola® and singing 'I'd like to teach the world to sing'. Today, there are many other global brands that enjoy similar status including Marlboro® cigarettes, Perrier® mineral water, McDonalds® restaurants and Levi's® jeans.

All of these global brands have emerged as part of the restructuring of the world economy (as discussed in Chapters 6–9). However, it is not simply the fact that more of us are drinking bottled water and wearing designer labels. In the context of this book, we need to explore how the rise of these brands is influencing our lifestyle choices, and thus our health, through their purveying of value systems, cultural identities and aspirations. To do this, we need to recognize that global brands do not happen by accident. They are created. In part, they are of course products that have a market. They would not become global unless there was widespread and significant demand for them. At the same time, such demand must be created, stimulated and encouraged by a whole army of marketing executives who design the advertising campaigns that make us want these products. And they have been very successful at doing this. Like the media giants described in Chapter 1, there are fewer and larger companies working to sell a broad range of products to markets around the world. Today, there are not many places in the world that you can go that has not been touched by the adman's hand.

Other cultural goods and services are being increasingly traded and thus contributing to global social change. According to the United Nations Educational, Scientific and Cultural Organization, trade in cultural goods has grown exponentially over the last two decades (Figure 2.2). Between 1980 and 1998, annual world trade of printed matter, literature, music, visual arts, cinema, photography, radio, television, games and sporting goods surged from US$95 million to US$388 million. Available data underestimates the boom in multimedia, audiovisual, software and other copyright based industries during the 1990s enabled by technological changes. For example, it is estimated that global retail sales of recorded music rose from US$27,000 million in 1990 to US$38,671 million in 1998. Figures cover sales in over 70 countries surveyed on an annual basis by the International Federation of the Phonographic Industry. The rapidly growing popularity of downloading music from the Internet, legally or otherwise, will render these figures grossly outdated.

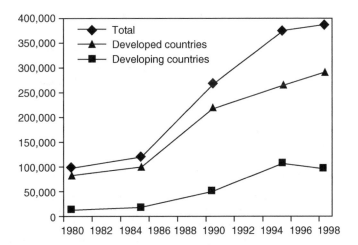

The US remains the largest exporter of cultural goods and services. In 1996, cultural products (films, music, television programmes, books, journals and computer software) became the largest US export, surpassing for the first time traditional industries such as automobiles, agriculture, aerospace and defence. Between 1977 and 1996, core copyright industries in the US grew three times as fast as the annual rate of the economy, achieving foreign sales and exports of US$60,180 million in 1996. Today Hollywood earns half of its revenues from overseas markets, compared to just 30% in 1980. Around 85% of worldwide screened films are currently made in Hollywood. In contrast, filmmakers on the African continent produced an average of 42 films per year, and are proportionally the largest importer of American films. Similarly, 95% of imported films in Chile and Costa Rica are American. Other industrialized countries are, to a lesser extent, major cultural exporters. In 1990, Japan, US, Germany and UK were the biggest exporters (55.4% of total exports), while the US, Germany, UK and France accounted for 47% of total imports. By the late 1990s, there were new players on the scene. By 1998 China has become the third most important exporter, and the new 'big five' were the source of 53% of cultural exports and 57% of imports (Figure 2.3).

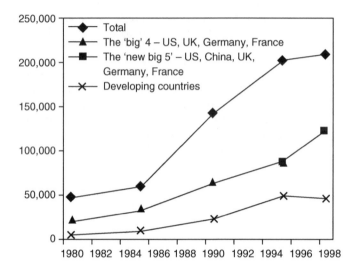

Activity 2.1

Look through your cupboards and make a list of around ten packaged store bought goods. Next to each item on the list, write the name of the company that has produced it. Try to identify if it has been produced by a locally owned company, subsidiary of a multinational company, or foreign-based company. How many products on your list can be described as 'global brands'? Think about the reasons why you decided to purchase each product? To what extent did marketing influence your decision?

Activity 2.2

For one week, compile a list of the advertisements you see around you (e.g. billboards, posters, signs) within your local community. What types of products do you see being advertised? How many products can be described as 'global brands'? Which products and type of products do you see most frequently advertised?

Health consequences of globalizing lifestyles and aspirations

There are undoubtedly many positive benefits arising from a growing trade in cultural goods. Cultures are never static, but continue to evolve and change over time. Nor is the use of advertising per se, of course, inherently wrong. Indeed, in principle, advertising has an intrinsic value by informing consumers about the characteristics of a product. This can foster competition among comparable products, forcing producers to improve on design, function or price. Advertising gives consumers a basis for selecting among these products available. Few would support the opposite extreme of products being wrapped in nondescript packaging and simply labelled (as formerly in some centrally planned economies).

Nonetheless, there are concerns, including health concerns, about the current imbalance in the source and content of cultural goods presently dominating contemporary crossborder flows. This is illustrated in the nature of advertising which has an ability, not only to guide consumption, but to shape it. The advertising of products harmful to health, such as tobacco, provides an obvious example. Figure 2.4 provides an example of how cigarette advertising can contain multiple messages. The advertisement is, of course, for cigarettes which are harmful to health. In addition, the imagery used to sell this product is noteworthy. The use of this glamorous image is intended to create certain aspirations, centred on its message that people (and particularly women) who smoke Virginia Slims are beautiful and successful. Chapter 9 describes the globalization of the tobacco industry and the pandemic of smoking-related diseases being created as a result. The effectiveness of this advertisement for selling cigarettes lies in its association of western imagery of glamour and beauty with smoking.

The widespread and growing use of skin lightening products is a good example of the power of the mass media to influence aspiration, resulting in adverse health consequences. In Africa, Asia, the Middle East, Latin America and the Caribbean, and among non-white ethnic groups in the US and elsewhere, large numbers of men, women and children use products containing steroids and the bleaching agent, hydroquinone (a white crystalline de-pigmenting agent), in an effort to lighten their skin colour. The products inhibit the production of melanin which naturally protects the skin against the harmful effects of the sun. Prolonged use of these products is leading to disfigurement, increased vulnerability to skin cancer, and mercury poisoning. The latter is known to cause neurological and kidney damage, and may lead to psychiatric disorders.

The reasons why such toxic products are so popular among non-white populations, despite their health risks, remain controversial. Local and historical associations between fair skin complexion and high social status (for example the wealthy do not need to work in the sun) clearly play a part. Yet most observers point to the ubiquitous presence of western culture, which has characterized contemporary globalization, as the main explanation. Even where images of non-white people are used in the mass media, there is a prevalence of 'Europeanized' ethnicity including relatively fair skin. For example:

> 'African ideals are increasingly based on images peddled by the white, Western world. Political liberation also brought an end to apartheid-era sanctions that had restricted foreign influences. But now South Africa's doors are wide open to

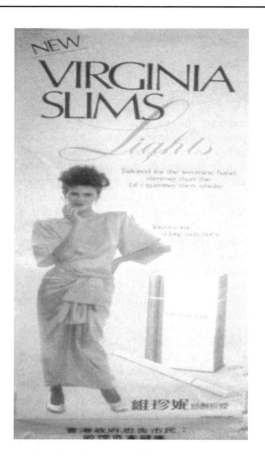

Western TV shows, movies, magazines, books – and values. The impact is unmistakable.' (Schuler, 1999)

'Media advertising worldwide greatly enhance the stereotypes that light skinned people are advantaged socially and romantically. In Jamaica, advertisements like these are not broadcast, printed or aired often, but the few depict light skinned women saying for example that "Vanishing Cream fades dark spots and freckles, lightens and brightens skin to a smooth radiant glow".' (Andrew, 2002)

'The culturally loaded issue today is the number of Asians looking to remake themselves to look more Caucasian. It's a charge many deny, although few would argue that under the relentless bombardment of Hollywood, satellite TV, and Madison Avenue, Asia's aesthetic ideal has changed drastically.' (Takeuchi Cullen, 2002)

This explanation seems to support related and rising trends among non-white populations in the use of hair straightening products, cosmetic surgery and eating disorders in the attempt to conform to this increasingly globalized beauty standard. Throughout the Far East, there has been an alarming boom in cosmetic surgery since the 1980s to make Oriental features more Caucasian. The most popular procedure is eye surgery (blepharoplasty) to create the 'double eyelid' characteristic of western faces. In 2001 1 million procedures were performed, double the number five years previously. In South Korea, it is estimated that one in ten adults have received such treatment. In Japan and South Korea, a procedure that severs the nerve in the calf muscle so that it will atrophy is intended to get rid of so-called 'radish-shaped calves'.

Among people of African origin, there is an increased use of liposuction to reduce the size of the hips and buttocks, and rhinoplasty to narrow and pointier the nose. As the sales director in South Africa for American Look hair straightening products described, 'In the [United] States, being African is hip right now. Here, people want to look American. They want to play basketball, drink Coke, and straighten their hair like Oprah Winfrey [a Black female talk show host]' (as quoted in Schuler, 1999).

Similar trends are beginning to be observed in the rising prevalence of dieting and eating disorders, notably among young people, notably women, in non-western countries. In Japan, it is estimated that one in 100 young women, and 5% of Tokyo junior schoolgirls, now suffers from an eating disorder, almost the same incidence as the US. The country is being flooded with imported diet aids, all of dubious efficacy and some even potentially dangerous, to feed the population's desire 'to get closer to the stick-like ideal represented by international fashion models and a growing number of their domestic idols' (Watts, 2002). As Efron (1997) writes,

> 'Over the past five years, the self-starvation syndrome [anorexia nervosa] has spread to women of all socioeconomic and ethnic backgrounds in Seoul, Hong Kong, and Singapore . . . Cases have been reported – though at much lower rates – in Taipei, Beijing and Shanghai. Anorexia has even surfaced among the affluent elite in countries where hunger remains a problem, including the Philippines, India and Pakistan'.

Seeking to understand how cultural context promotes the risk for eating disorders, a survey of Fijian adolescent girls was carried out one month and then three years after television was introduced to their local area. The study sought to understand the impact of novel, prolonged exposure to television on disordered eating attitudes and behaviours. The study found a negative impact from television, with the number of girls who practised self-induced vomiting to lose weight increasing from 0% to 11% between 1995 and 1998. Girls living in houses with television were three times more likely to show symptoms of eating disorders (Becker et al., 2002). A study of eating disorders in South Africa found a similar rise in incidence among young Zulu women. While 40% of the Zulu girls surveyed were overweight or obese, more than half had 'disordered eating attitudes and behaviours' including self-induced vomiting, and the use of laxatives and diet pills. The study reported that girls wanted to look less 'like their mums and more like western girls' (BBC News World Edition, 2002).

Research on the prevalence of eating disorders, and the causal factors contributing to their apparent rise within non-western countries, remain limited. As cultural globalization intensifies and embraces more communities, it will be important to better understand how this process takes place.

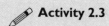

Activity 2.3

Obtain a copy of a popular women's magazine available locally. Look at the advertisements contained within it. What products do the advertisements seek to sell? What imagery of women is used to sell these products? Think about the discussion above and how these images might influence how young women perceive themselves.

Global social change and non-communicable disease

For many, the influence of cultural globalization is having somewhat different effects on lifestyle choices. It is now well recognized that there is a global rise in obesity taking place. Using the measure of body mass index (BMI), calculated by dividing an individual's weight (in kilograms) by height (in square metres), overweight is defined as BMI>25, obesity as BMI>30. The US, the most affluent country in the world, has led this trend. Results from a National Health and Nutrition Examination Survey (NHANES) for 1999–2000 by the US Centers for Disease Control and Prevention found an estimated 64% of adults are either overweight or obese. This represents an increase of 50% during the 1990s. Obesity is now responsible for 430,000 deaths in the US annually, second only to tobacco use, and consumes 12% of health care costs (US$117 billion per year). Of particular concern is the rapid rise in childhood obesity (Figure 2.5), with 15% of children and adolescents aged 6–19 years now overweight or obese (Ogden et al., 2002). These trends are predicted to have alarming public health consequences predicted in coming decades in the form of heart disease, diabetes and cancer.

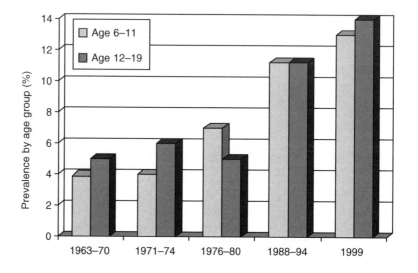

Importantly, the obesity epidemic is rapidly becoming a global issue. In other high-income countries, similar trends are beginning to be observed. Fifty per cent of European adults are now overweight, including an increase in obesity of 10–40% over the past ten years. Moreover, similar trends are beginning to be observed in many low- and middle-income countries. The International Obesity Task Force estimates that around 300 million people worldwide are obese. In India 30–40% of adults of high socioeconomic status are now obese. In China, where over-weight people are historically uncommon, the number of overweight people rose from 10% to 15% in three years. In Brazil and Colombia, the figure is around 40%. Even in sub-Saharan Africa, where undernutrition remains a problem for many, there has been an increase in obesity prevalence notably among urban women (Figure 2.6). Figure 2.7 illustrates the predicted trends in obesity for three countries by 2030.

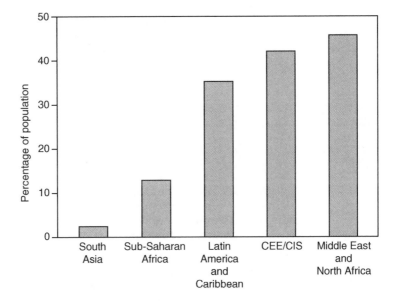

Explanations for these trends are undoubtedly complex, yet their widespread occurrence over a relatively short period of time, and their global occurrence, suggest a link with globalization processes. Changes to our patterns of energy intake and expenditure have been influenced by three key factors: the intensive marketing of unhealthy foods; lower production costs and thus greater use of oils, salt and sugar in food products; and the creation of living environments that discourage physical activity.

Of these three factors, the link between obesity and food marketing has so far received the bulk of attention. Much of the available evidence so far focuses on high-income countries. Explanations of the sharp rise in childhood obesity, in particular, has been attributed in large part to their increased exposure to marketing and advertising.

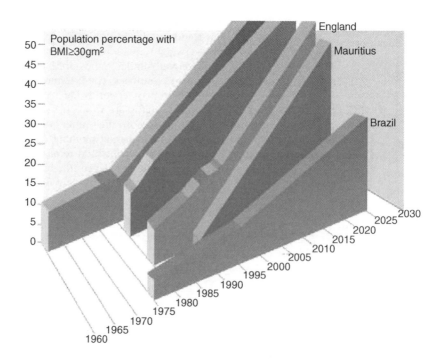

'During the same period in which childhood obesity has increased dramatically, there has also been an explosion in media targeted to children: TV shows and videos, specialized cable networks, video games, computer activities and Internet Web sites.' (Kaiser Family Foundation, 2004)

The average American child (2 to 18 years old) spends about five and a half hours daily using media including almost three hours watching television. In the US food is the second most advertised category of products (after automobiles). Marketing and advertising aimed at children increased from US$6.9 billion in 1992 to US$15 billion in 2002.

Evidence suggests that the spread of similar exposure to marketing in other parts of the world is contributing to the rise in obesity elsewhere. In 20 countries (including Germany, Israel and Greece), children watch more television than children in the US. In Mexico it is predicted that 6 million children will be using the Internet by 2004.

In his bestselling book, *Fast Food Nation*, Schlosser (2001) writes about the rapid rise of the fast food industry in the US and the psychology behind its popularity: 'Working-class families could finally afford to feed their kids restaurant food.' Playing on the natural parental desire to make their children happy, fast food restaurants collaborate with other global brands, such as Walt Disney, to play on this desire. He writes that parents 'want the kids to love them . . . It makes them feel like a good parent . . . only McDonald's makes it easy to get a bit of Disney magic.' The same advertising techniques and messages are being used to export fast food worldwide. Of particular concern is the amount of advertising targeted at children. McDonald's Restaurants, the most widely recognized brand in the world, spends more on advertising than any other brand. The franchise has 25,000 restaurants in 100 countries, with an average of five new restaurants opened each day. Eighty-five per cent of new restaurants now open outside of the US.

There is a growing move to more closely regulate marketing by the food industry, and particularly marketing targeted at children. In 2004 WHO published a report, *Marketing Food to Children: the Global Regulatory Environment* which reviews regulation of television advertising, in-school marketing, sponsorship, product placement, Internet marketing and sales promotions. In recent years, there has been increased regulatory activity surrounding television advertising, in particular, with proposals put forth in Australia, Brazil, France, Germany, India, Ireland, Italy, Malaysia, New Zealand, Poland and the UK (Hawkes, 2004). More directly, and reminiscent of the tobacco industry, legal cases have been brought against the food industry in the US and Brazil by litigants who hold food companies liable for adverse health consequences.

Should the food industry be held accountable for the looming pandemic of non-communicable diseases? This is the view of a growing number of lawyers, some of whom have provided legal representation against tobacco companies. The argument is that food companies use excessive amounts of salt, sugar and fat, and market those products in ways that people are encouraged to over consume. As Nestlé (2003) writes, 'many of the nutritional problems of Americans – not least of them obesity – can be traced to the food industry's imperative to encourage people to eat more in order to generate sales and increase income in a highly competitive marketplace'.

In Brazil a lawsuit was filed in July 2003 arguing that Coca-Cola and Ambev-Pepsi are culpable for the rising obesity rates in the country. The Consumer's Defence Public Attorney for Sao Paolo filed the suit to 'compel them [the companies] to stop advertising and marketing to children and to warn consumers about the risk of excessive sugar consumption'. The two cases are currently under appeal (Hawkes, 2004).

To stave off tighter regulation and potential litigation, 'Big Food' manufacturers have begun to modify their activities:

- Kraft Foods (owned by Philip Morris now known as Altria) has announced changes to the way it creates, packages and promotes its products including reducing portion size, fat content and caloric value of many foods.
- McDonald's Restaurants has introduced healthier alternatives to its menu including sliced fruit and salads.
- Frito-Lay (owned by PepsiCo) has committed to making at least half of its new food and beverage products for nutrition conscious consumers.

It remains to be seen whether these voluntary actions will be sufficient, whether companies will extend these changes to markets outside of the US, or whether, as is the case with the tobacco industry, double standards will operate.

Much remains to be understood about the precise causal mechanisms behind the rapid global rise in obesity rates, and the policy actions needed to tackle the problem. It is clear that the causal factors, and their consequences in the form of so-called 'lifestyle diseases', are increasingly global in nature. Recognizing this, in May 2004, WHO adopted a global strategy on diet, physical activity and health to 'reduce the risks and incidence of non-communicable diseases' worldwide. In doing so, WHO opened a new front in the battle to influence how we live within an emerging global society.

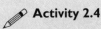 **Activity 2.4**

Keep a diary of the food you eat for one week. Think about what factors influenced your choice of diet. How readily available is fresh fruits and vegetables? How often did you eat processed and fast food products?

Summary

This chapter examined selected health implications arising from global social change, some of which will be considered in greater detail in subsequent chapters. Chapter 3 addresses the gender dimensions of globalization and health, while Chapter 4 describes the health impacts of globalization on the food industry.

References

Albrow M (1990) *Globalisation, Knowledge and Society*. London: Sage.

Andrew M (2002) 'The Skin Bleaching Phenomenon – Commentary,' 1 September 2002. Available at: http://www.jamaicans.com/cgi-bin/moxiebin/bm_tools.cgi?print=858; s=16_4;site=1

BBC News World Edition (2002) 'Eating disorders rise in Zulu women,' 4 November 2002. Available at: http://news.bbc.co.uk/2/hi/africa/2381161.stm

Becker A, Burwell R, Gilman S, Herzog D and Hamburg P (2002) 'Eating behaviours and attitudes following prolonged exposure to television among ethnic Fijian adolescent girls'. *British Journal of Psychiatry* 180: 509–14.

'Brief History of Tobacco Advertising to Women in Asia,' Speakers Kit on Women & Girls, Tobacco, & Lung Cancer, American College of Chest Physicians and The Chest Foundation, Northbrook, Illinois, no date. Available at: http://speakerskit.chestnet.org/wgtlc/index.php.

Compiled from US Centers for Disease Control and Prevention, National Center for Health Statistics, Table 69, 'Overweight children and adolescents 6–19 years of age,' 2003. Available at: http://www.cdc.gov/nchs/data/hus/tables/2003/03hus069.pdf

Dahlgren G and Whitehead M (1991) *Policies and strategies to promote social equity in health*. Stockholm: Institute for Futures Studies.

Efron S (1997) 'Women's Eating Disorders Go Global'. *Los Angeles Times*, 18 October 1997.

Hawkes C (2004) *The Global Regulatory Environment around Marketing Food to Children*. Geneva: WHO.

Huntington S (2002) *Clash of Civilizations and the Remaking of World Order*. New York: Free Press.

Kaiser Family Foundation (2004) 'The Role of Media in Childhood Obesity'. *Issue Brief*, February. Available at: www.kff.org.

Martorell R, 'Obesity' in 'A 2020 Vision for Food, Agriculture, and the Environment,' International Food Policy Research Institute (IFPRI). Available at: http://www.iotf.org/.

Nestlé M (2003) *Food Politics: How the Food Industry Influences Nutrition and Health*. University of California Press.

Ogden CL, Flegal KM, Carroll MD and Johnson CL (2002) 'Prevalence and trends in over-weight among US children and adolescents, 1999–2000'. *JAMA* 288: 1728–32.

Schlosser E (2001) *Fast Food Nation*. New York: Houghton Mifflin.

Schuler C (1999) 'Africans look for beauty in Western mirror'. *Christian Science Monitor*, 23 December.

Takeuchi Cullen L (2002) 'Changing Faces'. *Time Asia*, 5 August, 160(4).

UNESCO, *Culture, Trade and Globalisation, Questions and Answers* Paris: UNESCO 2000.

Watts J (2002) 'Japanese slimmers pay a high price for obsession'. *Guardian*, 2 August.

3 Gender, globalization and health

Overview

The pervasive nature of the economic and social impacts of globalization can be effectively illustrated by differentiating between men's and women's experiences of such change. A gender sensitive approach to public health can therefore valuably inform analysis of the multiple hazards and opportunities for health arising from globalization. This chapter analyses the links among gender, globalization and health, reviewing the impact of globalization on patterns of labour, distribution of wealth and social behaviour and highlighting their diverse implications for health. You will first learn about gender and health and then examine these concepts in a global context by looking at health reforms, globalization and trade, analysing their health impacts by focusing on poor women. It then examines the links among women's health, poverty and globalization with policy debates among multilaterals and the response of global health movements.

Learning objectives

After working through this chapter, you will be able to:

- **define gender and a gender perspective on health and globalization**
- **understand the debates around gender, health reforms, economic liberalization and health**
- **understand the links between poverty, gender and health**
- **understand the contribution of the health movement and the women's health and rights movement to global health policy debates.**

Key terms

Civil society Associations of citizens (outside their families, friends and businesses) entered into voluntarily to advance their interests, ideas and ideologies.

Gender A socio-economic variable with which to analyse roles, responsibilities, constraints and opportunities of men and women.

Gender perspective A gender perspective tries to discern the impact of gender in terms of structural (legal and economic), social (education, health and religious) and cultural mother, leader, carer dimensions.

Gender

Gender refers to differences between men and women that are socially constructed, changeable over time, and that have wide variations within and between cultures. Gender is a variable with which to analyse roles, responsibilities, constraints and opportunities of men and women.

Awareness of gender enables identification of inequalities between men and women. Such attitudes, or gender biases, are reflected in laws, policies and social practices, and in the self-identities, attitudes and behaviour of people. Unequal gender relations affect women's and men's choices in relation to health or employment and tend to deepen economic and social inequalities and discrimination based on class, race, age, sexual orientation, etc.

A gender perspective tries to discern such inequalities, whether they are structural, social or cultural. Gender bias may often go unrecognized, being viewed as something 'natural', as in the absence of women in decision-making bodies, awarding lower wages to women for equal work, or favouring boy children over girl children. Using a gender perspective to understand health is therefore essentially about analysing the different power relations, customs and norms that are reflected in almost all levels of life including systemic economic and political changes at the global level.

 Activity 3.1

Look through a national newspaper and see if there are any articles demonstrating an awareness of differences in the roles played by men or women. Look specifically for in-depth stories about particular economic or political activities. To what extent are women discussed at all in the articles?

 Feedback

Media coverage typically gives little attention to such issues, and any attention is usually confined to a section of a newspaper designated for women. As you progress through this chapter, think about the gender differences that underlie the stories you have selected and consider how such articles could incorporate gender.

Gender and health

Health is created in the context of everyday life and the gendered implications of health due to biology and social and economic factors can be felt at community and household level. There are clear differences in male and female patterns of health, sickness and death that are shaped by biological and social factors. Women's reproductive role makes them vulnerable to a wide range of health problems. Both women and men are susceptible to sex specific diseases such as cancers of the breast or prostate throughout their life cycle. For biological reasons there are differences in the vulnerability of women and men to diseases such as HIV-AIDS, heart disease and TB.

Women and men face different risks in terms of their health and well-being while also having differential access to resources that promote health. This is illustrated in the following extract from the International Women's Health Coalition (http:www.iwhc.org).

Women's vulnerability to HIV/AIDS: An overview

The combination of gender inequality and severe poverty is lethal to women in the developing world, and creates the following risk factors for HIV:

- Lack of comprehensive reproductive health services and information for women and girls. If the world community is serious about preventing transmission of HIV/AIDS in women, comprehensive reproductive health services should be a logical starting point for increased funding. But women's health education and services continue to be woefully underfunded.
- Economic disempowerment. Pressure to provide an income for themselves or their families leads many girls to engage in 'transactional sex' with older men ('sugar daddies'), who give them money, school fees, or gifts in exchange for sex.
- Lack of basic education. Of the 121 million children not in school worldwide, 65 million are girls, and the highest concentrations are in sub-Saharan Africa. AIDS is adding to the problem because girls are leaving school in increasing numbers, much more often than boys, to care for sick relatives. Education gives girls the skills they need to access information, enter the labour force, and rise above the poverty that makes them all the more vulnerable to infection.
- Migrant husbands. Many women, especially those in rural areas, are infected by husbands who work as miners, truckers, or soldiers and engage in unprotected sex while away from home. For example, in Cameroon, the HIV prevalence of men who have been absent from home for more than 31 days is 7.6%, compared to a rate of 1.4% among those who stayed home.
- Ignorance and stigma around HIV/AIDS. Widespread unwillingness to talk frankly about sex prevents the dissemination of accurate information about HIV/AIDS, fostering the spread of wildly inaccurate information. Often, the effects are especially harmful to women and girls, as in, the myth that having sex with a virgin can cure AIDS.
- Child marriage. In many developing countries young girls commonly marry before they are 18; 60% of girls in Nepal, 76% in Niger, and 50% in India will be married by that age. These young girls often know very little about sex, HIV, or how to protect themselves. Because they are so young, they have little power in the relationship, and so are unable to negotiate condom use. Additionally, girls and young women who are married are more likely to drop out of school.
- Violence. One in three women worldwide will be raped, beaten, coerced into sex, or otherwise abused in her lifetime. A woman who experiences sexual violence is at a physically greater risk of contracting HIV, and if she is in an abusive relationship, she is rarely able to negotiate terms to protect herself from infection.

Male and female patterns of health and illness are also influenced by other social factors. All societies assign gender roles to men or women. Men and women are expected to perform different duties and therefore have different entitlements to social and economic resources.

Broad changes associated with globalization have also had varying impacts on women's and men's health. Women and men have experienced differently the widespread health reforms altering access to health care and the capacity of women and men to control their sexual and reproductive lives; trade liberalization has led to different goods and products being available; and shifting patterns of waged and unwaged work have altered the distribution of resources.

The gendered effects of health reform

The 1980s and 1990s saw a shift in the international perception of health from a humanitarian issue to an issue of economic growth and security, bringing new political actors in the international health arena including the World Bank, the International Monetary Fund (IMF) and the World Trade Organization (WTO). Such actors have redefined health discourse epitomized by the World Bank's 1993 report 'Investing in Health Care'.

The report emphasizes two strategies. The first is the introduction of market forces into the health care sector and the allocation of public resources according to 'criteria of technical and instrumental efficiency'. The second is 'health care reorganization' or state withdrawal from the financing and provision of health services and a reorientation of public institutions toward selective assistance.

The main recommendation of the World Bank's health reforms was privatization of health care, to be understood as:

1 Introduction of user charges in state health facilities, especially for consumer drugs and curative care;
2 Promotion of third party insurance such as sickness funds and social security;
3 Promotion of private facilities and clinics; and
4 Decentralization of planning, budgeting and purchasing for government health services.

Health reforms in developing countries have resulted in cuts in public health services and the increased use of non-governmental and private voluntary organizations to deliver services. For example, 25% of hospital care in Ghana is private, in Zimbabwe 94% of services for the elderly are privatized, and in Uganda and Malawi 40% of all health services are privatized. Privatization has particularly reduced government funded primary care, thus limiting the access of poor women to health care. When poor women have to pay for health care, they typically do so for their children but not for themselves.

Gendered impacts of economic liberalization on health

Recent decades have seen major changes in the way goods and services are produced and a shift in women's and men's employment patterns. The global restructuring of production has been based on an increasing demand by employers for flexible labour that will meet their needs at the lowest possible cost. Many of the world's poorest women have entered the labour force, displacing male work, and disrupting traditional gender patterns in the work force and in the home.

These major shifts in the 1980s onwards has led to what many have called the 'feminization of labour' with millions of women taking on paid work in both formal and informal sectors. In 2000, women provided between 30% and 45% of the manufacturing work force in Latin America, Asia and Africa. In the export industries of South-East Asia, women make up over 80% of the workforce.

It can clearly be argued that increased access to waged work is good for health. An independent income enables women and men to buy what they need to promote their own health whether that is a better diet or a safe space to live. The workplace may also provide important social support, and women's access to jobs improves their self-esteem and bargaining power within the household. Increased employment opportunities can also give women increased mobility and enable access to primary and reproductive health care.

However for many women, particularly the poorest, gendered relations in the workplace and home can severely constrain the realization of these potential health benefits. Unskilled workforces associated with the feminization of labour have increased most rapidly in countries where regulatory regimes are weak and wages are low, exacerbating health hazards. Women's workloads (paid and unpaid) tend to increase with liberalization. If, for instance, women enter the workforce as 'additional workers' to offset the job loss of male household members, their work burdens may increase, they may lose leisure time, and their health and nutritional status may deteriorate. Male unemployment is also associated with gender-based violence, as described in the following extract from a UN declaration (1995):

Violence against women

'. . . violence against women constitutes a violation of the rights and fundamental freedoms of women . . .'

Preamble to the Declaration on the Elimination of Violence against Women . . . the first international human rights instrument to exclusively and explicitly address the issue of violence against women. It affirms that violence against women violates, impairs or nullifies women's human rights and their exercise of fundamental freedoms.

Article 1 of the Declaration . . . and the Platform for Action from the Fourth World Conference on Women (the Beijing Platform for Action) both define violence against women as:

any act of gender-based violence that results in, or is likely to result in, physical, sexual or psychological harm or suffering to women, including threats of such acts, coercion or arbitrary deprivation of liberty, whether occurring in public or in private life.

The Beijing Platform for Action commits governments around the world to take action to address violence against women. Among other demands, the Platform calls on governments to:

Condemn violence against women and refrain from invoking any custom, tradition or religious consideration to avoid their obligations with respect to its elimination as set out in the Declaration on the Elimination of Violence against Women;

Adopt and/or implement and periodically review and analyse legislation to ensure its effectiveness in eliminating violence against women, emphasizing the prevention of violence and the prosecution of offenders; take measures to ensure the protection of women subjected to violence, access to just and effective remedies, including compensation and indemnification and healing of victims, and rehabilitation of perpetrators;

Create or strengthen institutional mechanisms so that women and girls can report acts of violence against them in a safe and confidential environment, free from the fear of penalties or retaliation, and file charges;

Allocate adequate resources within the government budget and mobilize community resources for activities related to the elimination of violence against women, including resources for the implementation of plans of action at all appropriate levels.

Women mostly enter the labour force during their reproductive years, implying specific health concerns related to menstruation, pregnancy and breast feeding and care of children. This can put physical strain on women as well as psychological stress as women have had to search out new ways of meeting family needs without traditional sources of support. Some have been forced to migrate in order to find work or to avoid situations of conflict.

Gender, trade and health

Trade has a complex relation to gender and health, one that is just beginning to be analysed in detailed empirical studies that show both positive and negative health outcomes for men and women in poor countries. While removal of trade barriers may reduce the costs of imports such as food or contraceptives, costs may still be prohibitive for poorer households experiencing decreased incomes. There may be trade-related policy changes that operate through public expenditure and revenue generation that affect health. Trade liberalization affects government revenues through tariff reductions and other channels, which in turn may affect the allocation of public expenditure for public services, including expenditure for provision of primary and reproductive health care.

Trade agreements cover not only tariffs and quotas but also agricultural products, services, intellectual property rights, government procurement and overseas investment. Many agreements require countries to allow competition in health care, water, education and energy services, opening up the way for privatization and commercialization. These all have specific gendered impacts on poor people's health. While the health impacts of the World Trade Organization (WTO) will be discussed in more detail in Chapter 7, it is important here to highlight its often divergent effects by gender. The WTO's Agreement on Agriculture (AoA), for example, has been instrumental in liberalizing world agriculture. Commentators studying gender and trade have argued that such liberalization has worsened rural poverty, devastated agriculture and the livelihoods of poor farmers (the majority of whom are women) and deepened gender and class inequalities. The primary aim of the AoA is the increased production of cash crops, but such increases tend to benefit male farmers, and are often not passed on to their families. Many poor women farmers with the additional responsibility of looking after children, dependent elderly and relatives, are denied such benefits since they are engaged in agriculture for household or local consumption. The AoA thereby serves to undermine the security of household food with women bearing the brunt of having to secure livelihoods and food for their families. For example, large scale agriculture reform in the Philippines has led to a massive migration, largely of women from displaced families moving to find work in towns or overseas.

The privatization of drinking water, a major trade issue, directly impacts on the poor, particularly poor women because of their responsibilities in the household for sanitation and clean drinking water. As they are first in line in gathering and using water they are also more susceptible to water-borne diseases. Similarly, the impact of trade agreements in restricting access to medicine can impact disproportionately on poor women who typically take charge of their families health.

There are also concerns of the impact of the WTO on health and safety in the workplace. As women invariably have less skilled jobs, worse pay and working conditions, they are more likely to be exposed to health risks as well as job insecurity. Even in the service sector where women take up the majority of jobs and where pay and conditions are relatively better, women are still relegated to lower pay and have little health or other security. As the rules of the WTO's General Agreement on Trade in Services (GATS) push service liberalization, local providers are forced to compete with powerful transnationals, undermining working conditions and long term security.

Exposure to new hazards is especially common in factories in the Export Processing Zones in Asia and Latin America where women usually make up the majority of the workforce. In the case of the electronics industry for example, young women are often exposed to a multiplicity of toxic substances with chronic effects on both their physical and their mental health. However the greatest hazards probably face the many women in developing countries now exposed to the traditional hazards of old industries such as textiles.

The informal sector

Millions of women and men scrounge out a precarious living in the informal sector. The work is demanding, monotonous and physically debilitating. The sector is largely dominated by women.

> 'Most of the poor who are not involved in agriculture acquire their livelihoods in the informal sector . . . Much can be learnt from the work of the Self-employed Women's Association (SEWA) in India which focuses on organizing women in informal employment and is experimenting with schemes to provide health and life insurance to workers in the unregulated sector of the economy.' (Narayan, 2000)

Work, migration and health

Trade and economic liberalization is closely associated with large-scale migration. Many of the same countries that have opened up to trade in recent years have also had large-scale migration of labour from rural to urban areas. This has had a deeply gendered impact in South-East and East Asia. Migration can positively affect the health of women and their families. They may be able to move out of the family dominated social realm into a more public realm. Often, they have control over their earnings, even though they remit much of their earnings to their families. Movements into urban areas and to more developed countries can also bring greater access to health care.

Major difficulties can counter such positive impacts. Men and women workers can be highly exploited, but often women are particularly vulnerable due to gender bias. Migrants from Asian countries such as Indonesia or India to countries working in the Persian Gulf have few rights or access to services, often entering into demeaning contractual arrangements. Filipino domestic workers who migrate to Hong Kong and to the US, for example, often have a precarious legal status and may be under the control of their recruiting agent and employers, suffering long hours of work, unhygienic living conditions, sexual and physical abuse, and general vulnerability.

Migration can put women at greater risk of unwanted and unhealthy sexual activity. Without the protection of their home environment and in a new culture women can be exposed and exploited without the knowledge to defend themselves from sexual harassment or unhealthy sexual practices. Migrant men seeking sex put themselves and their sexual partners at risk of sexually related diseases in particular HIV/AIDS.

Gender, health and migration

The International Covenant on Economic, Social and Cultural Rights comments on the right to the highest attainable standard of health (Committee on Economic Social and Cultural Rights, 2000). This has been largely translated as a right to health *care* and has enabled a focus on ensuring that rights of individuals are not violated through the creation of structural and other barriers to the access of health care facilities. The approach has had some success with patients who are HIV positive, where stigmatization and discrimination have been particularly problematic obligations towards migrants and their health introduces a further challenge.

In 2000 the International Organization for Migration (IOM) estimated that there were 150 million people living outside the country of their birth. Globalization, conflict, environmental disasters have all contributed to the need for populations to be mobile. The marginalization and health of migrant populations is a growing public health concern as they represent one of the most 'at need' groups in the world. Compared to the dominant population of richer host countries they generally have worse physical and mental health outcomes and this has in fact been cited as a reason for restrictive immigration policies. There is a concern about the spread of communicable diseases; some that would be new to host countries if endemic in the countries of origin of the migrants, and others which are re-emerging, having been previously controlled, due to poor health and hygiene conditions in crowded refugee and internal displacement camps. In addition, some countries may reject applications for migration if a health problem is likely to impose a significant excessive cost on its health care system. Women migrants have a higher risk of being victimized in the workplace and subject to sexual exploitation and associated reproductive and mental health sequel. The health needs of migrant groups are often reflected in the high level of support required for healthy resettlement and 'integration'.

Poor women, health and globalization

Dr Gro Harlem Brundtland in 2000 stated that 'poverty has a women's face' – of the 1.3 billion of the poorest people 70% are women (UNDP, 1995). Therefore if you, as Dr Brundtland recommends, 'look at the world through the eyes and spirit of poor people' you need in particular to understand what 'health security' means for poor women.

The reduction of aid levels and public expenditure due to adjustment packages and subsequent debt servicing has led to severe deterioration of health services, equipment and facilities. These cuts have hit women both in terms of their own health and reproductive health needs and in terms of the heavier demands on their role as social producer. The health effects of the increasing poverty associated with these global trends has led to worsening maternal, infant and child mortality rates and a rise in communicable diseases.

Maternal mortality has increased by over 100,000 deaths since 1999. There are now an estimated 600,000 deaths a year due to pregnancy-related causes, 99% in low income countries. Even though in richer countries maternal mortality rates are almost negligible, many of the poorest countries have now the lifetime risk of one woman in ten or less dying from pregnancy-related causes (World Bank, 1997). Such figures may be under-reported given a reluctance to report maternal deaths. The impact of poor reproductive health can also be seen in the loss in disability adjusted life years (DALYs) (Figure 3.1).

The link of maternal mortality to economic and social changes is particularly marked in sub-Saharan Africa. When user chargers were introduced maternal deaths in the Zaria region of Nigeria rose by 56% along with a 46% decline in the number of deliveries in the main hospital. There is also evidence that introduction of fees has increased gender differences in health expenditure. For example, in Zambia expenditure on women's illness was less than a third than on men.

There are three particular areas where the link between poverty, women and ill-health has led to the increase in maternal mortality and decrease in poor women's health and well-being. First is the link between poverty, women and communicable disease due to the negative impacts of restructuring health reforms and privatization that globalization has exacerbated. Infectious disease emergence such as TB, malaria, HIV/AIDS has specific effects on poor women as gender and biology interact to produce greater vulnerability.

The second trend are the specific problems linked to new patterns of global consumption and distribution in the area of poverty and non-communicable diseases, food quality and nutrition that impact on women's health and also in their role as

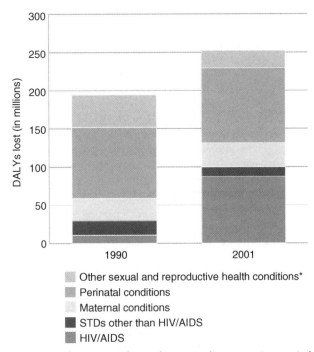

* Iron-deficiency anaemia for women of reproductive age; breast, ovarian, cervical and uterine cancer; and genitourinary diseases, excluding nephritis and nephrosis. Source: Singh, Darroch et al., 2004.

Figure 3.1 DALYs lost in women 15–44 due to sexual and reproductive health conditions

Source: UN Interim Report of Task Force 4 on Child Health and Maternal Health (2004) available at http://www.unmillenniumproject.org/documents/tf4interim.pdf.

carer of the family. Decreasing levels of nutrition, along with increasing obesity fed by marketing of unhealthy products combine with shifts in living conditions that threaten poor women's and their families' health.

Third is the critical issue of violence, now recognized as increasingly significant given the apparent rise in domestic and community violence, politically motivated fundamentalisms and escalation of national conflict. Women's movements and health NGO movement are not only dealing with the multiple impacts this violence has on poor women but have also successfully placed the issue on the international development agenda.

The Millennium Development Goals (MDGs) are a set of measurable benchmarks of national efforts to eradicate extreme poverty and hunger; achieve universal primary education; promote gender equality and empower women; reduce child mortality; improve maternal health; combat HIV/AIDS, malaria and other diseases; ensure environmental sustainability; and develop a global partnership for development. Health and gender in these goals are officially treated as cross cutting issues. In 2005 the Millennium Project task force reports provided recommendations to the UN Secretary General in the form of far reaching policy guidelines on how to achieve the goals.

The Preface and introduction of the Millennium Project Task Force on child health and maternal health 2005 states the following:

'What will it take to meet the Millennium Development Goals on child health and maternal health . . . by 2015? . . . The task force agreed on several principles from the very start. . . . [First] it requires wrestling with the power dynamics of power that underlie the patterns of population health in the world today. Second those patterns reveal deep inequities in health status and access to health care both between and equally important within countries . . . Moreover only a profound shift in how the global health and development community thinks about and addresses health systems can have the impact necessary to meet the Goals. . . . How can the power to create change be marshalled to transform the structures including the health systems that shape the lives of women and children in the world today?'

'. . . Women and children – a tag line for vulnerability, an SOS for rescue, a trigger for pangs of guilt. Change must begin right there. The Millennium Development Goals are not a charity ball. The women and children who make the statistics that drive the Goals are citizens of their countries and of the world. They are the present and future workers in their economies, caregivers of their families, stewards of the environment, innovators of technology. They are human beings. They have the rights – entitlements to the conditions including access to health care that will enable them to protect and promote their health to participate meaningfully in the decisions that affect their lives and to demand accountability from the people . . .'

 Activity 3.2

This is a highly political statement by a group of technical experts who are helping to set the direction of health policy to try and combat child and maternal mortality and morbidity through the intergovernmental system. How do you think an understanding of gender relations, health and globalization inform this debate?

Feedback

The report begins with the premise that health is a right for all, and that women and children are entitled to take up their rights, however poor, in whatever country. They see the potential for globalization working through the multilateral system to provide the means, resources and technical ability to reverse radically maternal mortality and morbidity, by ensuring women's right to quality prenatal and postnatal care. If governments were to value women's health the global networks, the resources and knowledge are in place for services, drugs, technical means to ensure that even the poorest countries can meet the MDG 5 to reduce by three quarters maternal mortality. What is required is a much stronger political support for the international conventions and agreements at that national level to create the enabling environment for women to space their children, for skilled birth attendance, proper referrals and in last resort emergency obstetric care. This requires economic and social change to provide distribution, resources and services for sexual and reproductive health and rights education, good maternal health care.

Globalization and health – civil society's response

As the effects of global restructuring have become more visible, many health groups have responded by becoming involved in political action. The most intensive campaigning has involved sexual and reproductive care and gender violence, needs-based campaigns relating to poverty and subsistence, occupational and environmental health as global restructuring has exposed both them and their families to new hazards.

Due to health reforms and the impact of trade and liberalization leading to states withdrawing funding for health care, the organizations making up 'civil society' have taken on greater responsibilities. Women have been especially active in this context with many moving from the role of volunteer service provider to community activist. At the same time, some of those entering the labour force have become involved in collective action to defend themselves against threats to their well-being.

Using new information technologies and deploying the universalizing framework of human rights they have highlighted the potential of 'virtual communities' in a globalized world. Despite major differences in material circumstances and socio-cultural identities they have worked together to promote more equitable gender relations as part of the wider campaign for a healthier world.

The 1978 concept of Primary Health Care (PHC) presented in the Alma-Ata Declaration of the World Health Assembly (2004). PHC was seen as the key strategy for achieving Health for All (HFA) by the year 2000. This strategy was based on the understanding that basic health care needs policies and programmes have to address the underlying economic, political and social disparities that lead to poor health. The principles that it encompassed were: 'universal access and coverage on the basis of needs; comprehensive care with an emphasis on disease prevention and health promotion; community and individual involvement and self reliance; intersectoral action for health; and appropriate technology and cost-effectiveness in relation to available resources.

The People's Health Movement (PHM) is an 'international network of organizations and individuals that came together in 2000 to re-ignite the call for Health for All Now!' The goal of the PHM is 'to re-establish health and equitable development as top priorities in local, national and international policy-making, with comprehensive primary health care as the strategy to achieve these priorities.' Its main aim is to begin with the work done by people's health movements around the world to develop long-term and sustainable solutions to health problems.

Towards this end, in December 2000 it held a People's Health Assembly (PHA) in Bangladesh. The PHA was a unique gathering. Unlike the WHO Health Assemblies this one involved people in village meetings, in district meetings, in national events, and in regional workshops to prepare for the global gathering in Bangladesh. The Assembly took place in a community health centre (GK) in Bangladesh where the accommodations were modest and where people had a chance to talk about their concerns regarding health. Over 1,400 people from 92 countries attended.

The preamble of the People's Charter for Health agreed in 2000, draws on the WHO/UNICEF Declaration on Primary Health Care agreed at Alma-Ata in 1978 to achieve Health for All. The Charter states: 'Health is a social, economic and political issue and above all a fundamental human right. Inequality, poverty, exploitation, violence and injustice are at the root of ill-health and the deaths of poor and marginalized people. Health for all means that powerful interests have to be challenged, that globalization has to be opposed, and that political and economic priorities have to be drastically changed. This Charter builds on perspectives of people whose voices have rarely been heard before, if at all. It encourages people to develop their own solutions and to hold accountable local authorities, national governments, international organizations and corporations.'

The following is from the People's Charter:

> 'Strong people's organisations and movements are fundamental to more demo-cratic, transparent and accountable decision-making processes. It is essential that people's civil, political, economic, social and cultural rights are ensured. While governments have the primary responsibility for promoting a more equitable approach to health and human rights, a wide range of civil society groups and movements, and the media have an important role to play in ensuring people's power and control in policy development and in the monitoring of its implementation.

This Charter calls on people of the world to:

49. Build and strengthen people's organisations to create a basis for analysis and action.
50. Promote, support and engage in actions that encourage people's involve-ment in decision-making in public services at all levels.
51. Demand that people's organisations be represented in local, national and international forms that are relevant to health.
52. Support local initiatives towards participatory democracy through the establishment of people-centred solidarity networks across the world.'

 Activity 3.3

How might a gender perspective be useful for understanding the challenges of fulfilling the Charter's aim of achieving health for all?

 Feedback

What is crucial about this movement is that women's issues are central to its charter and women's networks and activists are key actors and decision-makers in it.

It will be important to continue to keep this gender awareness in the campaigns building on the successes of the international women's health network. Some important gender dimensions to the campaign could be:

• including women as decision makers and leaders in the movement;
• building on women's networking experience particularly in relation to primary health care and reproductive and sexual rights and health;

- designing campaigns that take up women's and men's specific health needs for example in South Asia and Africa reducing maternal mortality, the need to bring HIV/AIDS firmly into the sexual reproductive rights and health campaigns;
- campaign to hold governments accountable to improving health services that take responsibilities for all areas of women's health throughout the life cycle.

Summary

You have learned about the relationship between gender and health and how this is influenced by globalization in terms of international economic forces and trade. You also have seen how the gender-health relationship is affected by other social determinants such as work, migration and poverty. Finally, you learned about civil society's response to these challenges.

References

Alma-Ata Declaration, Last Word (2004) Development Volume 47 No. 42 The Politics of Health, London: Palgrave Macmillan/Society for International Development.

International Women's Health Coalition (http:www.iwhc.org).

Narayan D (ed.) (2000) *Voices of the Poor*. Washington: World Bank.

UN Beijing Declaration and Platform for Action, Fourth World Conference on Women, 15 September 1995 A/CONF.177/20 (1995) and A/CONF.177/20/Add.1 (1995). http://www.un.org/womenwatch/daw/beijing/platform/.

4 The impact of globalization on food

Overview

In this chapter you will learn about the challenge of both under-nutrition and obesity globally, and the changes in the food chain that have occurred as a result of globalization and trade liberalization. You will then see how the increasing control of the food chain by agricultural and food corporations changes food security and diets.

Learning objectives

After working through this chapter, you will be able to:

- describe the global food security and under-nutrition situation
- describe the increasing public health challenge of overweight and obesity in low-, middle- and high-income countries
- sketch the food chain
- describe the increased significance of multinational and transnational corporations within this food chain
- understand how the changes in the global food chain are influencing diets

Key terms

Dietary changes Changes in the type and mix of foods consumed.

Dumping The placing of products in the international market at well below their production costs.

Food marketing The promotion of certain foods through the media and/or placement of vending machines in public places.

Food security The situation when all people, at all times, have physical, social and economic access to sufficient, safe and nutritious food that meets their dietary needs and food preferences for an active and healthy life.

Sustainable food supply A situation that ensures enough food of good quality, helps stimulate rural economies and promotes the social and environmental aspects of sustainable development.

Transnational corporation (TNC) A corporation that has developed coordinated control of its global business activities across national boundaries. This distinguishes the TNC from a multinational corporation (NMC), which operates in several countries but with limited coordination.

Introduction

In the context of food systems, globalization is nothing new. Trade in food has been documented since settled agriculture became the norm. This does not mean that the current phase is not qualitatively different. The sheer pace and scale of change is unprecedented. The global value of trading in food grew from $224 billion in 1972 to $438 billion in 1998; food now constitutes 11% of global trade, a percentage higher than fuel (Pinstrup-Andersen and Babinard, 2001).

For many the benefits from such an expansion in food trade have been great. Food production is at an all-time high having doubled in the past 40 years, as has production per capita. There is now more than enough food to feed everybody on the planet. Globally food prices have fallen by 50% and are at an all-time low (closely related to the huge US and European subsidies). Long-term forecasts indicate that prices are likely to remain low, at least in the medium term. This is reflected on supermarket shelves across the globe crammed with a cornucopia of different foods from different regions of the world. However there are a great many more people who are not benefiting from this state of affairs:

> 'FAO'S latest estimates signal a setback in the war against hunger. The number of chronically hungry people in developing countries declined by only 19 million between the World Food Summit (WFS) baseline period of 1990–1992 and 1999–2001.' (FAO, 2003)

This is the opening of the 2003 Food Insecurity Report illustrating the global failure to fulfil a basic right for millions of people. The reality is even worse than this. While there were reductions in the number of chronically hungry people in the first half of the 1990s, since 1995–97 the number has increased by over 18 million. Every day 799 million people in developing countries – about 18% of the world's population – go hungry. In South Asia one person in four goes hungry, and in sub-Saharan Africa the share is as high as one in three (FAO, 2003).

While hunger is difficult to measure, the situation regarding the proportion and numbers of people who are under-nourished is even bleaker. The number of under-nourished people actually increased by 4.5 million per year during the second half of the last decade. Twenty-six countries experienced increases in the number of under-nourished. Furthermore these countries were predominantly those that already had a large proportion of their population under-nourished (greater than 20%). Over the nine years from 1992 the number of hungry people in these countries increased by almost 60 million. The Millennium Development Goal of halving the percentage of hungry by half by 2015 is further away than ever.

When we focus more closely on childhood under-nutrition, as measured for instance by low weight for age, it appears that the situation in sub-Saharan Africa is particularly dire. While the goal of halving the proportion of underweight children has been achieved in South America, in Asia the drop in child malnutrition rates has been relatively small, from 36% to 29% (with China contributing to a large proportion of this), while in sub-Saharan Africa the proportion and absolute number of malnourished children has actually increased (Figure 4.1). Eastern Africa is the sub-region experiencing the largest increases in prevalence and numbers of underweight children – the number is projected to increase by 36% from 1990 to 2005. Findings for stunting, or extreme shortness of stature –

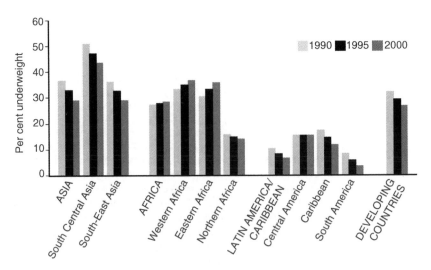

Figure 4.1 Trends in child malnutrition: developing countries, 1990–2000
Source: UNICEF, 2003.

which reflects long-term under-nutrition – and extreme thinness, or wasting, are similar.

Even more depressing is the lack of progress for women. According to the 5th Report on the World Nutrition Situation, out of the ten African countries with maternal nutrition data only three showed a decline in the prevalence of severe maternal under-nutrition (BMI<16) in the last decade.

The inevitable question is how can we explain this anomaly of increasing globalization resulting in increasing food production and cheaper prices but at the same time increasing numbers of under-nourished and hungry people?

 Activity 4.1

What may explain the paradox between increasing food production and increasing hunger worldwide? How might these reasons be linked to what you have learned so far about globalization?

 Feedback

Your answer may have included the growing evidence of the widening inequalities in income between the rich and poor. Differences in income distribution is in turn linked to differences in the distribution of food both between countries and within countries. This seems to be linked to many of the processes that are associated with globalization – liberalization of markets, increasing concentration of the ownership of land and capital, restriction in the movement of poor people versus the easier movement of capital, etc.

Over-nutrition

Over-nutrition and its associated risks of non-communicable diseases, including ischaemic heart disease, diabetes, stroke and hypertension, are usually perceived as a developed country problem. For example, recent surveys in the US have found more than half (55%) of the adults to be overweight and nearly a quarter to be obese (Flegal et al., 1998). Similarly, obesity levels have risen sharply in Europe albeit from lower levels. For example, the prevalence of obesity doubled to 16% in England from 1980–90 and is continuing to increase. This epidemic of obesity extols significant societal and personal costs in the forms of increased risk of disease and death, health care costs reduced social status, educational attainment and employment opportunities.

However, there is now increasing evidence that the problems of over-nutrition are growing rapidly in all parts of the world even in countries where hunger remains endemic. A number of recent reviews have shown significant increases in the prevalence of over-weight and obesity in developing countries. China is experiencing a rapid increase in over-weight and obesity in children and adults (Popkin and Doak, 1998). In countries such as Brazil and Mexico obesity is ceasing to be associated with higher socio-economic status and is becoming a marker of poverty, as is the case in developed countries. Some poor households in these countries are now suffering the double burden of under- and over-nutrition among household members.

Explaining the paradox

Understanding the impact of the globalization of agriculture and food systems on poor rural communities is critical if we are to make sense of the paradox outlined above. More than three-quarters of hungry people are in rural areas of developing countries. One in three live in rural landless and non-farm households such as those dependent on herding, fishing or forestry. One in every two suffering from hunger are in farm households on marginal lands, where environmental degradation threatens agricultural production. The situation for many of these peoples is worsening as poor fishers are seeing their catches reduced by commercial fishing, and foresters are losing their rights as logging companies move in under government concessions. Moreover, landlessness is rising in most rural regions because of higher farming densities and unequal land distribution. Average land per capita among rural farmers in developing countries declined from 3.6 hectares in 1972 to 0.26 hectares in 1992 – and stands to fall further by 2020.

You shall see later in this chapter how many of these changes can be linked to the impact of globalization on agriculture especially in developing countries.

✎ Activity 4.2

1 Draw a straight line horizontally across a piece of blank paper. Put the name of a foodstuff that you ate for dinner last night on the left hand end. Now write down on the right hand end the likely country of origin of the foodstuff. Then try to fill in as

many stages as possible the foodstuff might have gone through, from production to eventual consumption by you.

2 How do you think your food supply chain might be changing as a consequence of globalization? Have there be changes in recent years to the foods that you are able or not able to buy? Have there been changes in availability, quality, packaging, variety, sources or cost of certain foodstuffs?

Feedback

1 Your answer might look something like Figure 4.2.

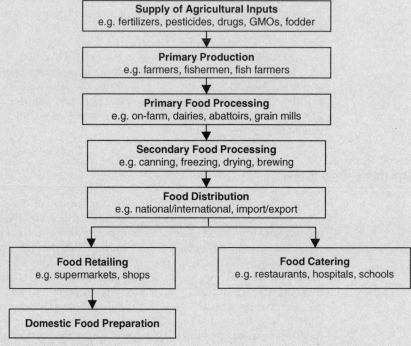

Supply of Agricultural Inputs
e.g. fertilizers, pesticides, drugs, GMOs, fodder

Primary Production
e.g. farmers, fishermen, fish farmers

Primary Food Processing
e.g. on-farm, dairies, abattoirs, grain mills

Secondary Food Processing
e.g. canning, freezing, drying, brewing

Food Distribution
e.g. national/international, import/export

Food Retailing
e.g. supermarkets, shops

Food Catering
e.g. restaurants, hospitals, schools

Domestic Food Preparation

Figure 4.2 The food chain

2 You may have noted some of the following changes

Increase in organic food – cheaper	Less home cooking
More local food but fewer local shops	Decline in food poverty
Province and prices	Variety diversity and availability
Scattered/fragmentation	Easier choice (labels and information)
Food technologies/food markets	Lower food prices
More specialized food markets	Allotments (land) for all
More supermarkets	Brand diminution and resistance

As you can see, the way in which food is grown, processed, distributed and marketed has changed dramatically just in the last 20 years. The example of wheat and livestock illustrates some of the more remarkable changes in each major part of the food chain and in particular their impact on diets.

Wheat: The New Deal price support programmes began to lead to large accumulation of surplus wheat in the United States after the Second World War. Through the Public Law 480 the United States was able to export to low income countries at concessional prices. Wheat exports grew 250% between 1950 and 1970 with low income countries' share increasing from 19% in the late 1950s to 66% in the late 1960s. In this period per capita consumption of wheat grew by 63% in low income countries while consumption of other cereals only rose by 20% and root crops fell by 20% in the same countries (Friedman, 1994).

This system allowed low income countries to cheaply feed an increasing urban working class and can explain some of the changes in diet associated with urbanization. For example, in Senegal a rural worker consumes about 158kg of millet, 19kg of rice and 2kg of wheat a year while his urban counterpart in Dakar consumes 10kg of millet, 77kg of rice and 33kg of wheat (Delpeuch, 1994). Further evidence for this comes from a FAO study that correlates levels of urbanization with imports of food (Table 4.1).

Table 4.1 Urbanization and food imports (study of 43 developing countries between 1970 and 1980)

Average increase in urban population as a share of total population	Average increase of imports as a proportion of total food available
1–5%	6.6%
5–10%	12.5%
>10%	14.8%

Data source: FAO, 1990.

The food crisis of the mid-1970s, by which time many countries were reliant upon wheat imports, saw the price of wheat rise dramatically and countries having to incur increased debt to pay for these imports. It also led to some countries such as Mexico, Columbia, India, Pakistan, Turkey and Argentina to switch over 80% of their total area planted in wheat to semi dwarf seed varieties, displacing rain-fed crops such as coarse grains, oilseeds and pulses. While this has allowed them to dramatically reduce their food imports it is at the expense of the more varied traditional crops usually cultivated for domestic production (McMichael, 1994).

Many other developing countries have not made this shift. The fastest growth of food imports has occurred in Africa which accounted for 18% of world imports in 2001 (up from 8% just 15 years previous to that). This has occurred partly because of a decline in agricultural and rural investment in Africa leading to a decline in agricultural productivity. Agricultural productivity per worker for the region as a whole has fallen by about 12% from US$424 in 1980 to an estimated US$365 per worker (constant 1995 US$) in the late 1990s (IFPRI 2004). Agricultural yields have also been level or falling for many crops in many countries. Significantly, yields of most important food grains, tubers and legumes (maize, millet, sorghum, yams, cassava, groundnuts) in most African countries are no higher today than in 1980. But the shift towards reliance of food imports has also occurred because of an acceleration of the 'dumping' of surplus cereals and foods from the United States and Europe:

'The Institute for Agriculture and Trade Policy have calculated that US subsidies are resulting in major crops being put on the international market at well below their production costs. Wheat by an average of 43% below cost of production; soya beans 25% below; cotton 61% below and rice 35% below cost of production.

This depression of commodity prices is having a devastating effect on farmers in developing countries. Research by the International Agriculture the International Food and Policy Research Institute (IFPRI) shows that subsidies to farming in the Organization for Economic Cooperation and Development (OECD) countries, which totalled US$311 billion in 2001 (or US$850 million per day), displaces farming in the developing countries, costing the world's poor countries about US$24 billion per year in lost agricultural and agro-industrial income. Moreover it is also hurting the farmers in the OECD countries as well as most of these subsidies go to the larger farms owned or contracted to corporations. For example, from 1997 to 2002, the US lost over 90,000 farms of below 2,000 acres, while farms above 2,000 acres increased by over 3,600.' (IATP, 2004)

'The World Trade Organisation does allow countries to block "dumping" of produce that is well below production price. But this mechanism, which can be costly and complex, is ironically mostly used by OECD countries. About one-half of anti-dumping actions are initiated against developing country producers, who take up to 8% of all exports. The use of anti-dumping actions by OECD producers, even when they are unlikely to win a dispute on its merits, creates onerous legal and other costs to current producers in developing countries, and chills new job-creating investment in sensitive sectors.' (IFPRI, 2003)

The potato is an example of the simultaneous transformation of diet and the globalization of agriculture. To ensure a steady supply of genetically standard fresh potato crops McCain re-organized traditional agricultural communities in Eastern Canada through monopoly contracts specifying most aspects of production and creating a monocultural region. At the same time the aggressive promotion of fried chips allowed McCains to generate large profits from frozen French fries before moving onto other high value-added products.

Livestock

The rise of the meat industry exemplifies many of the processes at play in the new food system. Meat production has doubled since 1997 and has increased five-fold over the last half-century. Since the early 1960s, the number of livestock has increased 60%, from 3 billion to more than 5 billion, and the number of fowl has quadrupled, from 4 billion to 16 billion. Producing meat requires large amounts of grain, and most of the corn and soy beans harvested in the world is used to fatten livestock. Producing one calorie of flesh (beef, pork or chicken) requires 11–17 calories of feed, so a meat eater's diet requires two to four times more land than a vegetarian's diet.

Three key factors have facilitated the explosion of meat production: a revolution in maize production based on hybrids requiring intensive mechanical and chemical inputs; substitution of forage crops by soya and a new capital-intensive feedstuffs industry that interposed itself between crop and livestock production. A globalized sector has emerged with global sourcing of feed inputs and global marketing of meat-related commodities. The whole system consists of a web of contractual relationships turning the farmer into a contractor, providing the labour and often some capital, but who never owns the product as it moves through the supply chain. If the poor are to benefit from the livestock revolution it will be 'by leaving mixed farming to specialise in livestock, and becoming contract farmers for food corporations in precarious dependency on distant markets and prices' (McMichael, 2001).

Concentration and power

A defining feature of globalization has been the increasing size and power of transnational corporations. In the agricultural industry this is reaching new levels. A few companies now dominate all parts of the food supply chain globally. To give a few examples in agricultural trade: six corporations account for 85% of world trade in grain, eight account for 60% of global coffee sales, seven for 90% of tea consumed in the West, three for 83% for world trade in coca, three for 80% of bananas (Madeley 2003). One TNC, Cargill, controls 80% of grain distribution throughout the world through its ownership of grain elevators, rail links, barges and ships (Kneen, 1996). The situation is the same in the agrochemical sector where ten agrochemical companies control 81% of the $29 billion global agro-chemical market; in Asia, three companies (Cargill, Pioneer and CP-DeKalb) currently control almost 70% of the seed market, supplying hybrid seed for 25% of the total corn area. Four corporations now own nearly 45% of all patents for staple crops such as rice, maize, wheat and potatoes (Action Aid, 2003). These TNCs have developed global brand names and have evolved global marketing strategies albeit with adaptation to local tastes. They are defined by the global sourcing of their supplies, the centralization of strategic assets, resources and decision making and the maintenance of operations in several countries to serve a more unified global market. For example, Hillsdown Holdings is now one of Europe's largest food conglomerates with a total of 150 subsidiary companies in Europe. It has important market share in such products as red meat, bacon, poultry and eggs. It also supplies the majority of its non-animal feed requirements from ten mills and its own chicks from its commercial hatcheries. Finally it has started to integrate downstream processing activities through the control of 25 abattoirs and several food processing, distribution and meat-trading companies (McMichael, 1994).

The manipulation and marketing of food

The challenge for the large food multinationals is how to increase profits when the food supply chain in developed countries is already completely saturated. The food supply contains 3,800 kcal for every adult and child in the United States (i.e. more than 150% of normal daily requirement). For many years now the prices of the raw agricultural products has remained stagnant or declined, the focus has thus moved towards increasing the profit margins further up the food supply chain towards processed foods. Processed foods and beverages are often referred to as 'value added' products, in that some combination of labour, technology and materials is applied to raw commodity inputs such as wheat and yeast, and transformed into a product such as bread or pastry. This is partly achieved through substitutionism. Substitutionism involves the progressive reduction of agricultural products to simple industrial inputs (which can be organic in origin) but allows replacement by increasingly non-agricultural components. Margarine, manufactured from cheaper intermediate ingredients as a substitute for butter, provides an early example of substitution; the rise of artificial sweeteners now accounts for more than half of US per capita consumption. In the United States, for example, 'farm' value has remained virtually unchanged in recent years while 'market' value (incorporating added value of the manufacture, retail and food services) has doubled and is now three times as large as farm value (Goodman and Watts, 1997).

You are now in a better position to understand the tendency of foods to be stripped of their nutritional content (as in white bread) and to be supplemented by chemical additives (such as colourings and flavourants). Sugar and salt are the two most commonly added ingredients with fats and oils also added in large doses to increase the 'added' value of foods (taking advantage of the biological fondness to sweetness and the easier to overcome satiety to sweet and fat foods). US, Western European and Japanese companies dominate the global food processing market. The 50 largest firms are located in these countries and account for roughly 40% of their gross output of manufactured food. In 2002 more than 11,300 new food products were introduced in the US alone.

Marketing of food

Coupled with the manipulation of foods has been the massive global marketing of foods. The food industry is the largest investor in global advertising. In the US alone the food industry spends over $30 billion on direct advertising and promotions. Food advertising is rising in developing countries as well – tripling in South-East Asia for example. Within a few years of their introduction, 65% of the Chinese population recognized the brand name of Coca-Cola, 42% recognized Pepsi and 40% recognized Nestlé (Lang, 2001). Mexicans now drink more Coca-Cola than milk. This shift in diet is accelerating as the food TNC's seek new markets. Global fast food and soft drinks companies have pursued aggressive international expansion strategies over the past few decades. Between 1991 and 2001, McDonald's more than doubled the number of countries of operation (from 59 to 121), more than quadrupled its number of non-US units (from 3,665 to 15,919), thus increasing its proportion of non-US outlets from 30 to 55%. Many developing countries have also developed their own versions of McDonalds.

Activity 4.3

Marketing activities can be classified into '5Ps':

- Place: the availability of the product (distribution) and location of sales points
- Price/package: the price of the product and its relationship with package
- Product expansion: creating and diversifying products

- Promotional activities: market entry marketing, advertising, sales promotions, websites
- Public relations: promoting the brand with good service; associating the brand with TV programmes, movies, sports, music and events, competitions and philanthropy

In your country, list the ways in which any fast food or soft drinks company are using the 5Ps to promote their product. Do you think these strategies are succeeding in changing the food choices of those around you?

But the dietary transition has also been explicitly encouraged through investments such as the World Bank's $93.5 million loan to China for 130 feedlots and five beef processing centres for its nascent beef industry and the entry of large food multinationals and food retailers into China. This moved Neal Barnard, president of the Physicians Committee for Responsible Medicine, to observe:

'While smart Americans recognize the need to "Easternize" their own diets with rice, soy products and more vegetarian options, World Bank bureaucrats decided to promote a Westernization of China's diet. Instead of supporting the use of grain as a cholesterol-free dietary staple for people, the grain will be fed to cattle to produce meat. Of course the World Bank's efforts to promote cattle farming in China are concerned less with good health than with economic investment. No doubt some cattle ranchers will profit, as they edge out vegetable and rice acreage. But why is the World Bank, so roundly criticized over for years for its self-defeating economic development schemes, falling into the same old trap?' (Quoted in McMichael, 2001)

This quote also draws our attention to the importance of the price and availability of foods that also influences dietary choices. Insightful studies from many settings have shown that high fat, high calorie diets are the most economical choices for poor people. It is therefore not surprising that the diets of poor people is dominated by cheaper fatty foods.

Summary

You have learnt how globalization is having a complex and often contradictory impact on diet and food security. One aspect is unequivocal: the increasing control by massive transnational corporations of all aspects of the food chain. Most low income countries are now reliant upon imports for food security with their domestic agriculture decimated by the sharp declines in food commodity prices internationally and the provision of cheap grains from the US and Europe. This in turn has dramatically changed the food preferences and diets of many in low income countries. Globalization is also having a profound impact on the diets of many either indirectly, through the availability of different foods or more directly through the marketing of certain types of foods. This would suggest that a more international public health response is required.

References

ActionAid (2003) *Going against the grain*. ActionAid.

Delpeuch B (1994) *Seed and surplus: an illustrated guide to the world food system*; translated by Chantal Finney and Alistair Smith. London: Farmers' Link.

FAO (1990) *Urbanisation and Food Systems*. Rome: FAO Publications.

FAO (2003) *The State of Food Insecurity in the World 2003*. Rome: FAO Publications.

Flegal KM, Carroll MD, Kuczmarski RJ and Johnson CL (1998) 'Overweight and obesity in the United States 1960–1994'. *Int J Obesity* 22(1): 39–47.

Friedman H (1994) 'Distance and durability: Shaky foundations of the world food economy'. In *The global restructuring of agro-food systems* (McMichael P, ed.). Ithaca: Cornell University Press.

Goodman D and Watts M (eds) (1997) *Globalising food: Agrarian questions and global restructuring*. London: Routledge.

Institute for Agriculture and Trade Policy (2004) *US dumping on world agricultural markets*. Minnesota: IATP, available on www.iatp.org (accessed 23 August 2004).

International Food and Policy Research Institute (2004) *How much does it hurt? Impact of agricultural polices on developing countries*. IFPRI, Washington DC, US available on www.ifpri.org (accessed 14 August 2004).

Kneen B (1996) *Invisible Giant*. London: Pluto Press.

Lang T (2001) 'Trade, public health and food'. In *International Co-operation in Health* (McKee M, Garner P and Stott R, eds) Oxford: Oxford University Press.

Madeley J (2003) *Food for all. The need for a new agriculture*. London: Zed Books.

McMichael P (2001) 'The impact of globalisation, free trade and technology on food and nutrition in the new millennium'. *Proc Nutr Soc.* 60(2): 215–20.

McMichael P (ed.) (1994) *The global restructuring of agro-food systems*. Ithaca: Cornell University Press.

Pinstrup-Andersen P and Babinard J (2001) 'Globalisation and human nutrition: Opportunities and risks for the poor in developing countries'. *African Journal of Food and Nutritional Sciences* 1: 9–18.

Popkin BM and Doak CM (1998) 'The obesity epidemic is a worldwide phenomenon'. *Nut Rev* 56: 106–14.

The impact of globalization on emerging infectious disease

Overview

In this chapter you will examine how globalization influences both the impact of human infectious diseases and the response to them. You will consider how globalization increases the interdependence of different countries, and what this means for the spread and control of infections. This is followed by a discussion of efforts to strengthen cooperative responses to infectious disease threats by the public health community. This includes an analysis of the main institutional players and the policies which they have supported.

Learning objectives

After working through this chapter, you will be able to:

- recognize the historical context of global threats from infectious disease
- understand the concept of emerging infections and the role of globalization in contributing to this growing risk
- describe corresponding changes in the concept of populations at risk, and how this modifies existing approaches to the control of infections
- be aware of the developing response by the public health community to the increasingly global threat from infectious diseases.

Key terms

Emerging infection An infection that has newly appeared in a population, or has previously existed but is rapidly increasing in incidence or geographic range.

Population at risk A population subgroup that is more likely to be exposed or is more sensitive to an infection than is the general population.

Quarantine The practice of isolating an individual who has or is suspected of having a disease, in order to prevent spreading the disease to others.

The history of population movements and infectious disease control

The threat from infectious diseases posed by the movement of populations has long been recognized. As long as the human species has migrated from one physical location to another, so too have microbes. For example, it is believed that smallpox was spread to Europe for the first time between AD 165 and AD 180, carried across the Roman Empire by troops returning from the Parthian Wars in Mesopotamia. During the third century, it is believed that bubonic plague began to move from its place of origin, along the Himalayan borderlands between India and China, to Egypt and Libya on the back of burgeoning trade between the regions. By the sixth century, bubonic plague reached Europe for the first time (Plague of Justinian of AD 542), commencing a cycle of plague lasting until the middle of the eighth century. A second cycle occurred eight centuries later (infamously known as the Black Death), killing between a quarter and half of affected populations. It was this epidemic that led to the development of quarantine as a means of preventing the spread of infection. This entailed ships arriving from infected ports to remain anchored for 40 days before being permitted to land.

Throughout the history of epidemics, the tension between effective disease control, and the free movement of people and trade, has been a key feature (Revision of the International Health Regulations, 1999a). A lack of scientific knowledge, as well as capacity to enforce public health measures, also hampered the prevention and control of outbreaks. One successful example began in September 1665 when plague came to the English village of Eyam, Derbyshire, probably via fleas in a box of cloth brought from London. The villagers, realizing the threat they posed to the surrounding communities, went into voluntary quarantine. In turn, residents of the surrounding area left provisions on the village boundary. During the year the village remained in isolation, about 260 people (one-third of the population) died. In other cases, such as on crowded ships without refrigeration or effective methods of preservation, the temptation to subvert quarantine measures by lying or sailing to a port where regulations were less stringent, was enormous. As a result, quarantine enjoyed limited success as a form of international health cooperation.

The first International Sanitary Conference (ISC) took place in Paris in 1851 at which participants sought to agree standardized quarantine regulations for the prevention of the importation of cholera, plague and yellow fever. Progress remained impeded by a lack of understanding of the mode of transmission of infection. Notably, the British delegate did not think that John Snow's new theory that cholera was transmitted by faecally contaminated water, worthy of mention. Furthermore the British were concerned to protect their primacy in international trade, and that the real purpose of increased regulation was to interfere with the flow of goods. The convention failed to produce agreement, but did establish that improved exchange of information about infectious disease outbreaks should be addressed internationally.

The development of modern microbiology and the revolution in understanding communicable disease, during the second half of the nineteenth century, laid the foundation for improved international mechanisms to prevent the spread of communicable disease. Improvements in public health at national level in some countries were paralleled by awareness of international aspects of communicable disease control. These developments were largely driven by European concerns over the threat of cholera from Asia. At the fifth ISC held in 1881, a proposal was made to create a permanent International Sanitary Agency of Notification. While this body was never created, due to a lack of support from participating governments, an International Sanitary Bureau (later the Pan American Sanitary Bureau) was established in Washington in 1896, along with the *Office International d'Hygiene Publique* (OIHP) in Paris in 1907. The OIHP considered the development of common standards for biological products, and for reporting health statistics, as among its main responsibilities, presaging the work of the World Health Organization.

After the First World War, the creation of the League of Nations in 1919 included in its Covenant that members would 'endeavour to take steps in matters of international concern for the prevention and control of disease'. The need for such cooperation was underscored by the 'Spanish' influenza pandemic of 1918–19 which is estimated to have caused between 20 million and 40 million deaths. The origins of the worst pandemic in history are uncertain, but it is clear that returning soldiers from the front, as well as mass migration, directly contributed to the spread of the disease (Oxford, 2002; Potter, 2001). Despite the scale of the outbreak, the US government decided not to join the League of Nations, thus undermining the formation of a single international health organization. Instead, three separate organizations, the Pan American Sanitary Organization (PASO), the existing OIHP in Paris, and a new Health Committee of the League co-existed until after the Second World War.

The World Health Organization (WHO) was created in 1948 to unify international health cooperation within a single body. Communicable disease surveillance was within the remit of the new organization from the outset. Another influenza epidemic in 1947 stimulated closer cooperation between national laboratories and public health authorities, resulting in the development of national and international reference laboratories for influenza. The success of this model was then extended to the development of a network of WHO collaborating centres.

Importantly, WHO became responsible for the International Health Regulations (IHR), binding on member states regarding cholera, plague, yellow fever and smallpox (later removed following global eradication). The purpose of the IHR is to 'ensure the maximum security against the international spread of diseases with a minimum interference with world traffic'. Almost immediately, however, there was considerable anxiety that the IHR was not achieving their stated aims. Critics argued that the regulations were rigid and inflexible, and could not be used to counter new or unknown infections. Moreover, the surveillance infrastructure needed for compliance was not in place in many countries, permitted prevention measures were perceived as excessive, and there was a widespread lack of compliance. In recent years, efforts to revise the IHR have been undertaken, with the aim of enhancing the timeliness and appropriateness of reporting international outbreaks (Revision of the International Health Regulations, 1999b).

Activity 5.1

What are the current limitations of the International Health Regulations in relation to globalization and infectious diseases?

Feedback

Your response should recognize that the original IHR only apply to cholera, smallpox, plague and yellow fever. They do not provide a legal framework for other infectious diseases including threats from emerging infections. Nor do the IHR allow for intervention before there is a clear diagnosis of the disease concerned. Finally, the enforcement of the IHR remains dependent on the cooperation of governments and there are no resources to ensure compliance such as punitive measures.

Under the auspices of WHO, a number of major programmes on communicable disease control were developed which required collaboration among countries and institutions. Some of these initiatives, such as the programme to eradicate smallpox, were spectacularly successful. Much collaboration was carried out through centres of microbiological and virological expertise, focusing on standards for biological reagents, test materials and procedures. Developments in surveillance tended to lag behind developments in laboratory skills. While international surveillance teams assisted in the investigation of particular problems, longer-term surveillance structures, with the regular interchange of data about communicable disease between those with responsibilities in surveillance and control, were not developed. Reporting to WHO for publication in the *Weekly Epidemiological Record* was a useful exercise for analysis of long-term trends, but not for public health action.

Globalization and emerging infectious diseases

Infection results from the interplay of a host, a pathogen and their environment. There is growing evidence that globalization may be affecting each of these factors, in turn, impacting on both the epidemiology of certain infections, and the required response to them. The focus of this section is on emerging infections defined as an infection that has newly appeared in a population, or has previously existed, but is rapidly increasing in incidence or geographic range (Table 5.1). New and emerging infections can result from changes in the host such as interventions which produced immuno-compromised individuals; in the pathogen such as the development of antimicrobial resistance; or in the environment such as global warming leading to changes in the range of insect vectors (see Chapter 10).

The link between globalization and emerging infections is most directly linked to changes in the environment in which host and pathogen interplay. Most notably, perhaps, the increased mobility of populations both in scale and geographical reach is believed to be increasing the likelihood that an infectious disease outbreak may involve more than one country. Some 2 million people cross international boundaries each day. The conditions created by this large-scale movement of people, other life forms, and traded goods around the globe, are also conducive to the movement of organisms and vectors (often insects) of disease. This can lead to the spread of infections to new areas where neither previously existed. In the shorter term, previously unaffected populations are at greater risk from new infections. In the longer term, the pooling of organisms may reduce the possibility that there are large populations completely naïve to particular organisms. A good

Table 5.1 Some major emerging infectious diseases

Organism	Transmission	Reason(s) for emergence
Borrelia burgdorferi	tick bite	Increased deer and human populations
Campylobacter jejuni	contaminated food, water or milk; faecal-oral	Increased recognition; consumption of uncooked poultry
Chlamydia trachomatis	Sexual intercourse	Increased sexual activity
Clostridium difficile	Faecal-oral; environmental contamination	Increased recognition; immunosuppression
Crimean-Congo hemorrhagic fever	tick bite	increased exposure to ticks
Cryptococcus	Inhalation	Immunosuppression
Cryptosporidium	Faecal-oral, person-to-person, waterborne	Development near water areas; immunosuppression
Dengue	mosquito bite	Poor mosquito control; increased urbanization; increased travel
Ehrlichia chaffeensis	Unknown? tick	Increased recognition; increase in host and vector pop.
Escherichia coli O157:H7	Ingestion of contaminated food	? a new pathogen
Filoviruses (Marburg, Ebola)	contact with infected blood, body fluids	Unknown; virus-infected monkeys shipped
Giardia lamblia	Ingestion of contaminated food, water	Inadequate water supply; immunosuppression; international travel
Haemophilus influenzae biogroup aegyptius	Contact with discharges;? eye flies	? increase in virulence due to mutation
Hantaviruses	Inhalation of rodent urine and faeces	Increased human contact with rodents
Helicobacter pylori	contaminated food or water, esp.; infected pets	Increased recognition
Hepatitis C	contaminated blood or plasma; sexual transmission	Recognition; blood transfusion practices
Hepatitis E	Contaminated water	Newly recognized
HIV-1/2	blood or body fluid; vertical transmission	changes in lifestyles/mores; intravenous drug use; international travel; medical technology (transfusions/transplants)
Human herpesvirus 6 (HHV-6)	Unknown;? respiratory spread	Newly recognized
Human papillomavirus	Direct contact	Newly recognized; ?changes in sexual lifestyle
Human parvovirus B19	respiratory secretions; vertical transmission	Newly recognized
Lassa	urine or faeces of infected rodents	Increased rodent infestation
Legionella pneumophila	Air-cooling systems, water supplies	Increased recognition
Mycobacterium tuberculosis	Droplet inhalation, reactivation	Immunosuppression

Table 5.1—*continued*

Organism	Transmission	Reason(s) for emergence
New variant CJD	Exposure to Bovine spongiform encephalopathy (BSE) agent	?Changes in the rendering process allowing agent into cattle feed
Nipah Virus	Droplet spread	Contact with animal reservoir, New agent?
Plasmodium	Mosquito bite	Urbanization; environmental changes; drug resistance; air travel
Pneumocystis carinii	Unknown;? reactivation	Immunosuppression
SARS Agent SARS related coronavirus	? droplet – person to person,? faecal – oral	Contact with animal reservoir, New agent?
Toxoplasma gondii	Cat faeces	Immunosuppression; increase in cats as pets

Source: *Emerging Infections: Microbial Threats to Health in the United States* (1992). http://www.nap.edu/openbook/0309047412/html/199.html.

example is the increase in so-called 'sex tourism', a controversial trend whereby relatively wealthy individuals from high-income countries travel to weakly regulated poorer countries to exploit the economically disadvantaged. Gillies (1992) found that 25% of those attending a genito-urinary medicine clinic, who had travelled in the previous three months, reported a new sexual partner while abroad. While sex tourism has become economically important for many communities, the communicable disease consequences from HIV/AIDS and other sexually shared infections are considerable.

Globalization can also impact on the broad determinants of health which make certain populations more or less vulnerable to infections. This includes influences on levels of household income and employment opportunities which can be highly differential. In some areas, economic globalization can bring development, growth and thus increased resources for health. For other populations, globalization has brought increased poverty, employment insecurity and deterioration in living conditions, thus increasing the risk of infectious disease. In many parts of the developing world, rapid urbanization means that when outbreaks do occur they are likely to be larger as the populations exposed to any event are likely to be larger. Current policy debates over the relative balance between the winners and losers from economic globalization are discussed in Chapter 6.

Other links between globalization and infection are becoming clearer. Deforestation, land clearance and migration are outcomes of global economic changes, and is increasingly associated with the emergence of infection. One example is the outbreak of Venezuelan haemorrhagic fever. Deforestation has probably been critical to the development of conditions which enabled the emergence of the infection. Migration into the area, followed by new settlements, led to increasing contact between humans and rodent hosts of the virus (Tesh, 1994). Other examples include the increased incidence and distribution of Yellow fever infection (Bryan, 2004), and the production of conditions conducive to mosquito breeding and transmission of malaria. Malaria can be reduced by land clearance as local mosquito habitats are destroyed, or may be increased as a result of bringing individuals into endemic areas, or altering the insect vector population (Molyneux, 2003).

There is also substantial debate about the extent to which globalization undermines or facilitates public health responses to communicable disease control. Critics of economic reform policies advocated by the World Bank and International Monetary Fund (IMF) since the 1980s, collectively known as structural adjustment programmes (SAPs), argue that resultant cuts in public spending has undermined public health infrastructure. This has included immunization programmes with consequent deterioration in the control of infectious disease. For instance, an outbreak of cholera in South Africa in August 2000, resulting in 46,000 cases and more than 100 deaths, has been attributed to the introduction of water charges, as part of the government's structural adjustment programme, in KwaZulu-Natal (McGreal, 2001). With around 80% of people having no running water or toilets, the epidemic quickly spread among rural dwellers. Similarly, the Asian economic crisis in 1997–98, and the consequent rise in poverty in the region, was seen to undermine global efforts to control the spread of tuberculosis.

 Activity 5.2

Look at the list of emerging infections in Table 5.1. It provides an overview of emerging diseases over recent decades. Select one of the diseases on the list and consider how its emergence might have been influenced by changes brought about by globalization.

 Feedback

The change in the epidemiology of each of the diseases will be different, and in most cases multifactorial. You should consider changes in host behaviour (such as sexual mores), changes in the agent (such as mutations leading to antimicrobial resistance or increased virulence), and changes in the environment (such as deforestation or a collapse of vector control). Each of these may have been influenced by such factors as the international sex trade, global marketing of antibiotics, large scale logging of primary forests, or the price of insecticides.

Developing global responses to emerging infectious diseases

Recognition that globalization may be impacting in a myriad of ways on infectious diseases including emerging infections, has led to efforts to develop effective global responses. One important development has been the development of global surveillance networks. Surveillance remains fundamentally a local activity, given that data needs to be collected at local level, and action needs to be taken as close to the origin of an outbreak in time and space as possible. Even an international outbreak can only be controlled through local action to control a source or sources and spread. For example SARS was controlled through concerted local efforts to identify and isolate infectious, or potentially infectious, individuals. Collaboration was required so that the actions of one country did not harm other countries' efforts to control the outbreak, such as by withholding information. Cooperation was also needed to ensure that international efforts were coordinated to best effect, for example, in the rapid identification of the new coronavirus causing SARS.

While the response to a global infectious disease threat needs to be built upon effective local surveillance and control measures, this does not mean that there is no value in regional and global responses. Indeed, it might be argued that an effective response to a disease threat arising from the globalizing world is necessarily through a globalized response. The evolution of the European Community, for example, encompassing the liberalized movement of goods and services, and increasingly labour, is perhaps an exemplar of the trends to globalization. This increasingly close union has brought both threats and opportunities in relation to communicable disease control. The increased awareness of possible outbreaks involving more than one country, and the necessity to coordinate investigation of such events, has stimulated discussion over the most appropriate mechanism(s) for facilitating and developing communicable disease surveillance at the European level.

 Activity 5.3

List the population at risk for the following events:

- an outbreak of meningitis at an international youth football tournament;
- an outbreak of *E. coli* from the consumption of an internationally traded foodstuff; and
- an outbreak of Legionnaires' disease among visitors to a hotel at a major holiday resort.

How might disease prevention, control and treatment systems be strengthened globally to respond effectively to these situations?

 Feedback

You should have considered the population at risk as all those who may have been exposed to the source. For example, people are at risk who have consumed the foodstuff and who may have travelled to other countries. There may also be secondary contacts to track down who may also be located in other countries. Early information about the source and who has been exposed (e.g. were all the cases at the football match staying in one hotel?) will help to focus interventions. Timely data collection requires sufficiently strong public health infrastructure, and effective action requires good communication systems to inform those responsible for taking action. When multiple countries are involved, this requires common standards of reporting, investigation and intervention.

An example of international cooperation is the European Working Group for Legionella infections (EWGLI) formed in 1986. Members are scientists with an interest in improving knowledge and information on the clinical and environmental aspects of Legionnaires' disease through developments in diagnosis, management and treatment of the disease. Legionnaires' disease is a potentially serious pneumonia caused by the bacteria *Legionella pneumophila* which thrives in conditions found in inadequately maintained air conditioning systems and spa baths such as Jacuzzis, where a spray of water is formed which may be inhaled. Outbreaks are often associated with leisure facilities such as hotels. Guests staying in a hotel, which proved the source of an outbreak of Legionnaires' disease, may be residents of several different countries. In 1987 the group established a surveillance scheme (known as EWGLINET), which detects cases of Legionnaires' disease in people who developed the disease as a result of staying in hotels or other types of holiday accommodation. The scheme aims to rapidly identify outbreaks so that control measures to prevent further cases can be taken, and the source of infection investigated. The goal of EWGLI members is to protect European citizens from the risk of developing Legionnaires' disease as a result of travel, either in their own country or abroad.

While existing mechanisms for communicable disease control depend heavily on government institutions, shortfalls in capacity and/or willingness to collaborate during outbreaks have remained a key challenge. In the past, many countries where a serious disease outbreak has occurred have faced major economic consequences. These include the cholera outbreak in Peru during the early 1990s, plague in Surat, India in 1993, and the crisis over variant Creutzfeldt-Jakob disease in the UK throughout the 1990s. In all three cases, substantial economic costs were borne by the affected country as other countries restricted trade and travel. In doing so, perverse incentives are created which make it less likely that a country will admit to a problem, and will try to manage an outbreak without alerting other countries. The slow reporting of the SARS outbreak by the Chinese government in 2002 is likely to have reflected concerns about the economic impact of such a revelation.

The only international regulations for the control of infectious disease remain the IHR which, as discussed above, is inadequate for the task and currently under revision. It has been suggested that more effective regulations would ask countries to send an alert when faced with a public health problem that might become of international concern. Countries should alert WHO on clinical suspicion, and not wait for microbiological confirmation. Importantly, countries who act as good citizens should be supported in controlling the outbreak, and be reassured that other countries are prevented from taking measures that lead to undue economic consequences for the affected country.

Finally, while globalization creates new risks, it also offers new opportunities for enhancing communicable disease response. Foremost is the potential to facilitate disease surveillance and reporting through more extensive and rapid communication. This is evident in the development of global networks for communicable disease surveillance and response such as ProMed and GOARN (Gouvras, 2004).

✎ Activity 5.4

A variety of regional and global networks for communicable disease surveillance now exist. Most are available electronically or printed form. Some examples are Euro-Surveillance (www.Eurosurveillance.org and *EuroSurveillance Monthly*), PACNET (Pacific Health Network), and the *World Epidemiological Review*. Think about why these networks have been developed in recent years. What benefits are such networks likely to provide in terms of local, regional and global public health action? What kind of information do you think would be useful to exchange across countries? In what ways do you think globalization might be used to improve infectious disease prevention, control and treatment?

 Feedback

Your answers should consider how information contributes to the different components of global disease surveillance, prevention and control. Globalization may provide the stimulus for alignment of practice between different jurisdictions. Globalization can also offer better communication tools for professionals.

Summary

You have examined how globalization may be influencing human susceptibility to certain infectious diseases, and the need to rethink institutional responses to them. Foremost is the way in which globalization is increasing the movement of people and infectious agents across national borders, as well as changing the social and natural environment within which people live. As you will learn later in this book, infectious diseases raise fundamental challenges for the development of global health governance.

References

Bryan CS, Moss SW and Kahn RJ (2004) 'Yellow fever in the Americas'. *Infect Dis Clin North Am*, 18(2): 275–92.

Emerging Infections: Microbial Threats to Health in the United States (1992) Institute of Medicine (IOM), Washington. Available at http://www.nap.edu/openbook/0309047412/html/199.html.

Gillies P, Slack R, Stoddart N and Conway S (1992) 'HIV-related risk behaviour in UK holiday-makers,' *Aids*, 6(3): 339–41.

Gouvras G (2004) 'The European Centre for Disease Prevention and Control'. *Euro Surveillance*, 9(10).

McGreal C (2001) 'Cholera township clear out stirs apartheid memories,' *Guardian*, 14 February.

Molyneux DH (2003) 'Common themes in changing vector-borne disease scenarios'. *Trans R Soc Trop Med Hyg*, 97(2): 129–32.

Potter CW (2001) 'A history of influenza'. *Journal of Applied Microbiology*, 91(4): 572–9.

Revision of the International Health Regulations (1999a) 'Public Health and Trade. Comparing the roles of 3 international organisations'. *WER*, 25: 193–201.

Revision of the International Health Regulations (1999b) 'Progress Report'. *WER*, 30: 252–3.

Tesh RB (1994) 'The emerging epidemiology of Venezuelan hemorrhagic fever and Oropouche fever in tropical South America'. *Ann N Y Acad Sci*, 740: 129–37.

6 Introduction to the global economy

Overview

In this chapter you will be introduced to economic globalization defined in terms of changes taking place to trade and finance. You will learn about three key institutional actors governing the emerging global economy – World Bank, International Monetary Fund (IMF) and World Economic Forum. Finally, the ongoing debate over whether globalization is good or bad for health is reviewed in relation to available evidence on economic growth, poverty and equity.

Learning objectives

After working through this chapter, you will be able to:

- define three types of economic globalization, and the shift from an international to a global economy
- understand the role of the World Bank, IMF and World Economic Forum in governing economic globalization
- describe the key debates on the positive and negative health effects of economic globalization.

Key terms

Economic globalization The process by which flows of goods and services, capital, labour or other means of production and exchange cross, and increasingly circumvent, national borders.

Global economy An economy whereby production, exchange and consumption are not linked to territorial distances but transcend national borders (transborder).

International economy An economy whereby production, exchange and consumption take place across national borders (crossborder) between entities located in two or more countries.

Three types of economic globalization

You can begin by distinguishing between two main components of economic globalization – trade and finance. Trade concerns the way in which goods and services are produced and exchanged between different countries. The globalization of trade means that there has been a *quantitative* increase in goods and services flowing among countries, as well as a *qualitative* change in the way they are produced. The globalization of finance concerns the increased quantity of currency trading, banking (savings and credit) and investment among countries, as well as a qualitative change in how financial transactions are carried out. In both trade and finance, in other words, what we are seeing is both a greater intensity of flows occurring across countries, and a greater number of countries involved in these flows.

Scholte (2000) identifies three types of economic globalization taking place (Table 6.1). Distinguishing among them helps to clarify frequent debates about whether globalization is occurring or not, the extent to which it is happening, and its timeframe.

Table 6.1 Three types of economic globalization

crossing of borders (internationalization)	increased crossborder movements between countries of people, goods, money, investments, messages and ideas
opening of borders (liberalization)	progressive removal of border controls
transcendence of borders (globalization)	patterns of production, exchange, and consumption become increasingly delinked from geography of distances and borders

Source: Scholte, 2000.

Crossing of borders is what most people commonly refer to as economic globalization. This occurs when the production of a good or service takes place in Country A, and is then exported to consumers in Country B. For example, a South African factory may produce medical equipment in Cape Town. It could then export this equipment to hospitals in other African countries and elsewhere in the world. This type of crossborder trade can be termed *internationalization*.

Trade between people across vast distances has taken place throughout human history (e.g. the Silk Route). When the modern system of states was formed in the seventeenth century, trade relations became more complex. Trade boomed over the next two centuries as goods and services, capital and even labour (e.g. slavery) were exchanged worldwide as part of the Industrial Revolution. Indeed, some writers argue that levels of crossborder trade (relative to total gross national product) actually rivalled the levels of trade we see today. People moved about without passports, trade flourished across continents, and the world economy grew rapidly. In this sense, it is sometimes argued that 'globalization', in the form of crossborder trade, is not new.

The latter two types of economic globalization, however, suggest that something distinct appears to be happening. The opening of borders, or trade *liberalization*, has accelerated rapidly since 1945. In the years leading up to the Second World War, many countries adopted policies that protected domestic industries and inhibited international trade. This worsened an already depressed world economy and contributed to the outbreak of war. The most powerful countries came together in 1944 in Bretton Woods, US to create three institutions that hopefully would prevent this happening again – the World Bank, IMF and General Agreement on Tariffs and Trade (GATT). The health implications of trade liberalization will be covered in Chapter 8. It suffices to say here that trade liberalization has led to the progressive removal of border controls, encouraging international trade to flourish.

The third type of economic globalization concerns the transcendence of borders, what Scholte (2000) defines more strictly as *globalization*. This describes how flows of trade and finance have come to circumvent, and even ignore, geographical space (notably national borders) so that they take on a new economic logic. Various writers have described this transcendence of borders by which the globe becomes the scale of operation. For example, in his book *Global Squeeze*, Longworth (1998) describes the Caterpillar plant in Toronto which does not manufacture heavy machinery but rather assembles winches from Brazil, engines from Japan, axles from Belgium and transmissions from the US. The final product is then exported worldwide. Similarly, as you learnt in Chapter 4, food production has been increasingly broken down into stages – from basic foodstuffs to consumption – located in different geographical locations. The entire chain of production might be overseen by a single company which might be responsible for product development, marketing and distribution to consumers.

As well as goods and services, economic globalization means the transborder flow of finance. Indeed, financial markets are evolving to support globalized trans-actions. Perhaps the most significant event in the emergence of a global financial system has been the so-called 'big bang' of the late 1980s which was, in fact, a series of policies adopted to liberalize and deregulate the financial sector. It was a key event in the emerging global economy because it enabled currencies, credit, investments and other financial assets to flow across the world with less attention to geography. Today, about US$1.5 trillion travel across borders daily as foreign exchange transactions.

The following quote about Dutch bank ABN-AMRO is taken from one of the bank's brochures: 'ABN-AMRO is one of the world's largest banking groups. Established in 1824, when King William I founded the Dutch Trading Company, today it has over 3000 branches in 60 countries and boasts 15 million customers worldwide.' (ABN-AMRO Bank, 2005)

Thousands of individuals choose to invest in specialized funds under its manage-ment. Many funds are global in reach, with fund managers buying shares in companies around the world. There is a lot of buying and selling as the company tries to earn the best return from different companies around the world. Multi-ply this activity millions of times over and you get a sense of what is happening to investment worldwide. Money handed to a financial advisor joins a global system that truly transcends borders.

One of the investment funds that ABN-AMRO offers is its Global Emerging Markets Fund whose investment objective is, 'To achieve long-term capital appreciation by investing in transferable equity securities of companies in emerging markets worldwide.' Its top ten holdings in June 2004 were as follows (Table 6.2):

Table 6.2 ABN-AMRO's top ten holdings

Company	Sector	Country	% of assets
Samsung Electronics	information technology	South Korea	7
Anglo American plc	resources	UK	3.5
SK Telecommunications	telecommunication	South Korea	3.1
America Movil SA	telecommunication	Mexico	2.9
Standard Bank Group	financial	South Africa	2.4
Vimpel Communications	telecommunication	Russia	2.3
Teva Pharmaceutical	pharmaceutical	Israel	2.3
Petroleo Brasileiro	energy	Brazil	2.3
Lukoil Holdings	energy	Russia	2.2
Gazprom	energy	Russia	2.1

Source: ABN-AMRO Bank (2005).

The scale of crossborder financial transactions between 1980 and 1995 has accelerated, with the value of world stock exchanges increasing 970% and value of foreign exchange transactions increasing 2,100% during this time (Anderson and Cavanagh, 2000). Liberalization of financial flows by governments around the world has encouraged such flows of capital, outpacing growth in world trade at 440% during the same period.

There remains much debate about the timing of the global economy's emergence, and extent to which it is happening. Available evidence suggests that economic globalization is taking place in certain sectors like pharmaceuticals, food, tobacco, textiles, automobiles, electronics and some service sectors. In other sectors, such as health care, it may only be happening to a limited degree. So it is more accurate to describe the world economy as 'globalizing' rather than 'globalized'. Some sectors lend themselves to being 'globalized' because they don't require one geographical base, or may benefit from production based across different geographical locations. Others may remain heavily regulated by national authorities and are not, and may never be, fully untied from physical geography.

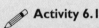 **Activity 6.1**

Look at a copy of a national newspaper in your country or a major newspaper available internationally such as the *International Herald Tribune, New York Times* or *Le Monde*. Ensure that the newspaper has a business section.

1 Scan the business section and see what proportion of the stories is concerned with local companies versus global corporations.
2 Can you identify examples of businesses which carry out operations in more than one country? What parts of the production chain are carried out where? Where does the company source and process raw materials? Where are the company's major markets for its product(s)?

Who are the big players in the global economy?

Important evidence of an emerging global economy is the growth in large corporations, from around 7,000 in the 1970s to over 50,000 in the late 1990s. Definition is important here. The terms multinational corporation and transnational corporation are often used interchangeably.

In talking about economic globalization, we need to distinguish between the two. A *multinational corporation* (MNC) remains headquartered in a home country, and then sets up subsidiaries in other countries. Subsidiaries may replicate the parent company's operations but primary decision-making power remains at headquarters. A *transnational corporation* (TNC) is qualitatively different, with operations structured to support a decentralized pattern of production and exchange as described above. Hence, different parts of the production chain may be located in different parts of the world.

A globalizing world economy means, not only that there are more TNCs, but that these companies are becoming more economically powerful. Today, certain industrial sectors are dominated by only a few very large companies, many of them commanding resources comparable to entire countries. Figure 6.1 shows that Exxon Mobil is the largest company in the world with annual revenues of over US$200 billion. This is larger than the GDP of Turkey and Austria. Similarly, the US retailer Wal-Mart has annual revenues of around US$190 billion.

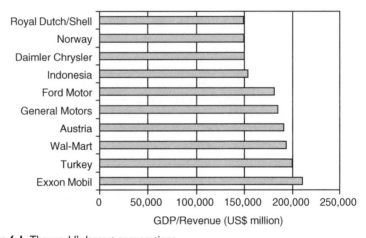

Figure 6.1 The world's largest corporations

Source: Compiled from Anderson S and Cavenagh J. http://www.ips-dc.org/downloads/Top_200.pdf.

If profits, rather than annual revenue, is argued to be a fairer measure of size, Table 6.3 shows that Exxon Mobil is also the most profitable company in the world with almost US$18 billion in profit (2000), a 124% increase over 1999. Other highly profitable sectors in the emerging global economy are electronics, banking and communications. Among the products these companies produce, many have direct health relevance.

Key institutions governing economic globalization

How did we get to where we are today? Has this happened naturally, as neoliberal economic theorists would argue, by allowing market forces to find efficiencies

Table 6.3 Corporations with the highest profits (2000)

Corporation	Profits (2000) US$ million	% change in profits from 1999
Exxon Mobil	17,720	124
Citigroup	13,519	37
General Electric	12,735	18
Royal Dutch/Shell	12,719	48
BP	11,870	137
Verizon Commun.	11,797	180
ING Group	11,075	110
Intel	10,535	44
Microsoft	9,421	21
Royal Philips	8,874	362

Source: Compiled from *Fortune*, 23 July 2001.

through greater economies of scale within and across countries? Can we see the growth and rise of larger corporations as the result of an economic 'survival of the fittest' within a competitive world market, and therefore a positive trend that should be encouraged? Some writers argue that the 'invisible hand' of the market is rationalizing economies worldwide. Economic globalization, in this sense, is seen as the triumph of capitalism writ large, a progressive force driven by basic economic laws. And like boats rising with the tide, it is argued that all will benefit ultimately from these trends.

However, many critics of economic globalization dispute this explanation, arguing that these processes are the result of deliberate policy decisions, then embedded within powerful institutional structures and rules of governance. This perspective sees globalization as a set of processes driven by certain vested interests and ideological principles which have, in turn, defined the nature and direction of economic globalization today. Foremost is the creation of clear winners and losers by globalization.

It is beyond the scope of this book to describe in detail all the relevant institutions concerned with governance of economic globalization. However, a basic understanding of the World Bank, IMF and World Economic Forum provides an important starting point for understanding how the world economy has come to be structured as it is today. The World Trade Organization (WTO) is addressed in Chapter 7.

While the roots of the world economy date back centuries, events leading up to and after the Second World War institutionalized the main principles and practices that define economic globalization today. A key factor contributing to the outbreak of war in 1939 was the world economic crisis. Beginning with the crash of stock markets known as Black Thursday (29 October 1929), followed by the worst economic depression in world history, country after country tried to protect its domestic economies by putting up higher trade barriers. This 'tit for tat' or 'beggar thy neighbour' policy effectively worsened the situation across the world, contributing to worldwide economic downturn.

The harsh lessons from these events led world leaders to create a new economic order that would ensure stability, trade and economic growth. A conference was held in Bretton Woods, US to create the institutions that would govern this new world economy.

World Bank

The World Bank was created initially to support the rebuilding of economies devastated by the war. Financed and governed by its member states, its initial role was defined as providing loans to countries for basic infrastructure such as dams, roads and power plants. Backed by major governments, the Bank proceeded to borrow funds on commercial markets with interest, and then re-loan these funds to applicant countries at a slightly higher rate of interest to ensure a return. There was a need for the World Bank because it could provide loans to countries that may not have been able to access the commercial market at such competitive rates.

There are five Bank institutions with the following functions:

- to provide 'soft loans' at low or no interest to poorest countries (International Development Association);
- to support private sector investment in Bank-approved projects (International Finance Corporation);
- to provide risk insurance to foreign companies seeking to invest in member states (Multilateral Insurance Guarantee Agency);
- to settle financial disputes among member states (International Centre for Settlement of Investment Disputes); and
- to provide low-cost loans for economic development purposes (International Bank for Reconstruction and Development).

The latter is the branch most commonly referred to as the World Bank. For health development purposes, the IDA is also important because it provides medium- to long-term loans at very low interest to the poorest countries.

Formally, the World Bank (along with the IMF) is a specialized agency of the UN system, but it has historically acted separately. This is reflected in its membership and decision-making process. The World Bank consists of member states who can take part in decision making. But, unlike other UN specialized agencies that are ruled by the 'one state, one vote' principle, voting rights are based on a member state's financial contribution. Under this rule, the world's ten richest countries hold around 54% of the votes, with the US holding the largest share (17%). In contrast, 48 sub-Saharan African countries hold around 5% of votes. The Bank is headed by a Board of Governors which is comprised of all 184 member states. Beneath this, and where the real power lies, is a select group of 24 member states (Board of Executive Directors) that make key decisions (Figure 6.2). The Bank is managed by an elected President who customarily is an American citizen. Four Managing Directors also oversee operations, along with over 11,000 staff in 100 offices in 181 member states. Staff are organized by Vice Presidential Units (VPUs) including six regional vice presidencies and seven thematically based networks. Health experts are based in regional units and networks (notably Human Development).

The World Bank's importance to economic globalization stems from its capacity to lend considerable sums to ministries of finance (around US$20 billion per year). As a lender of last resort, the Bank has the power to require governments to adopt certain policies in order to receive a loan. Since the early 1980s, policy conditionality has focused on making national economies 'leaner and meaner', under so-called

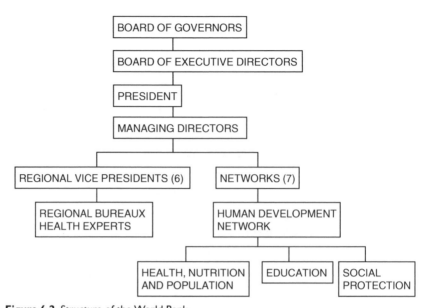

Figure 6.2 Structure of the World Bank

Source: Compiled from data collected from http://www.worldbank.org/.

structural adjustment programmes (SAP), and to integrate them with an emerging global economy. It was held that if countries strengthened private markets, supported trade liberalization, and encouraged foreign investment, economic growth would bring benefit to all. Almost immediately, however, such policies were criticized for failing to take sufficient account of their wider social and environmental consequences. Accumulating evidence from a wide variety of contexts suggested adverse health effects:

- In Costa Rica, a 35% cut in health programmes under a SAP was followed by a dramatic increase in infectious disease rates and infant mortality.
- In South Africa, the introduction of water charges under the SAP is believed to have led to a serious outbreak of cholera in eastern KwaZulu-Natal in 2001.
- In Peru a SAP was adopted following the debt crisis in the early 1980s. Between 1975 and 1985 estimated food intake declined by 25%. The further adoption of an IMF-led 'Fujishock' in 1992, which led to a significant decline in health expenditure and introduction of user fees, is blamed for a serious cholera outbreak.
- In China the introduction of user fees for tuberculosis treatment resulted in some 1.5 million cases being left untreated, leading to an additional 10 million people becoming infected (Werner and Sanders, 1997).

Despite criticism, the World Bank remains one of the institutional pillars of economic globalization. Cognizant of the concerns levied against it, there have been efforts to give greater attention to poverty reduction and social capital as important development goals. Nonetheless, debates remain about the nature of the loans it provides, the conditionalities attached, and the structure of decision making that governs its activities.

International Monetary Fund

The International Monetary Fund (IMF) was created to improve the financial stability and predictability of the world economy. Its role was to manage international flows of finance, acting as a foreign exchange facility for international trade. Its specific functions are:

- to facilitate the expansion and balanced growth of international trade, and contribute to the promotion and maintenance of high levels of employment and real income;
- to oversee a system of fixed exchange rates (preventing countries from devaluing national currencies to gain a trade advantage);
- to promote currency convertibility; and
- to act as lender of last resort through emergency loans to resolve short-term cash flow problems.

These functions were generally supported by the international community given the clear need for an effective mechanism for solving short-term imbalances in national economies. However, criticisms of the IMF have been similar to those levied at the Bank, namely its governance structure and, relatedly, appropriateness of its policy conditions. The IMF is governed by a Board of Governors, the highest decision-making body of the organization, consisting of one Governor (usually minister of finance or equivalent official) and an Alternate from each of the 183 member states. A 24-member Executive Board is delegated responsibility for conducting the business of the IMF, chaired by a Managing Director. The Managing Director, the chief of operating staff, is selected by the Executive Board and is customarily a European citizen. The number of votes that a member state holds is commensurate with the size of its quota (special drawing rights), allocated according to the country's economic ranking. The five countries with the largest quotas can appoint their own Executive Director, along with the two largest creditors. The remaining board members are elected by member states.

The weighting of decision making in the IMF in favour of the most economically powerful has been widely criticized. Of particular concern has been the organization's ability, like the World Bank, to make lines of credit conditional upon the achievement of economic stabilization and structural reform objectives. Like the Bank, it has promoted neoliberal-based economic principles with varied effects at best. These principles, summarized as a set of policy ideas known as the Washington Consensus (because many of the institutions behind them are based in Washington DC) are:

- Fiscal discipline
- Redirection of public expenditure
- Tax reform
- Financial liberalization
- Single competitive exchange rate
- Trade liberalization
- Elimination of barriers to FDI
- Privatization of state-owned enterprises
- Deregulation of market entry and competition
- Assurance of secure property rights

(Williamson, 1990)

Again, such policies have focused on trade and growth, with less attention to broader social and environmental needs. While the IMF will remain a key institutional player in managing economic globalization, its record in handling recent crises (e.g. Asian financial crisis of 1997), and widespread calls for its reform, make it likely that its role will continue to evolve.

World Economic Forum

The World Economic Forum (WEF) describes itself as 'an independent international organization committed to improving the state of the world. The forum provides a collaborative framework for the world's leaders to address global issues, engaging in particular its corporate members in global citizenship.' Boasting membership of over 1,000 leading companies and 200 smaller businesses, it is difficult to dispute its status as 'the foremost global community of business, political, intellectual and other leaders of society'. The WEF holds a wide range of regional and international meetings, with the most well-known being its annual meeting in Davos, Switzerland which brings together around 2,000 'of the most knowledgeable, dynamic and influential people in the world' from more than 100 countries. Health initiatives include a Global Institute for Partnership and Governance, a platform to launch private-public partnerships.

Criticisms of the WEF focus on its élitist membership. A regional breakdown of its 1,007 organizational members (Table 6.4) reveals a transnational class of political and economic élite who dominate contemporary globalization. As an alternative forum, NGOs have held a World Social Forum since 2001 to challenge this élite 'to listen to the needs and concerns of poorer communities and an opportunity for campaigners from across the globe to meet' (Christian Aid, 2002).

Table 6.4 Organizational members of the World Economic Forum by region

Region	No. of members	% of total
Europe	430	43
North America	262	26
Asia	131	13
Central/South America	75	7
Middle East	45	4
Africa	43	4
Australasia	22	2

Source: compiled from data on WEF website: www.weforum.org.

In summary, the World Bank, IMF and WEF are important pillars of current forms of economic globalization. Achieving good governance of this emerging global economy remains a key challenge. There will be continued debate whether these institutions (reformed or otherwise) should form part of global economic governance, or whether alternative institutions need to be created.

Activity 6.2

How does the WEF differ from the World Social Forum (WSF) in terms of purpose and participation?

Feedback

The stated purpose of the WEF contrasts with the World Social Forum (WSF) which describes itself as 'an open meeting place for reflective thinking, democratic debate of ideas, formulation of proposals, free exchange of experiences and inter-linking for effective action, by groups and movements of civil society that are opposed to neo-liberalism and to domination of the world by capital and any form of imperialism, and are committed to building a society centred on the human person'. However, participants are not called on to take decisions as a body, whether by vote or acclamation or declarations or proposals for action that would commit all, or the majority of them. Rather, it is open to pluralism and to the diversity of activities and ways of engaging of the organization and movements that decide to participate in it, as well as the diversity of genders, ethnicities, cultures, generations and physical capabilities.

Is economic globalization good or bad for health?

The great debate surrounding economic globalization concerns its true impacts on people's lives, and in particular, the lives of poor people around the world. This is a highly polarized debate, and lies at the heart of so-called anti-globalization demonstrations. The key dispute is whether the emerging global economy, as currently structured and directed, is a positive or negative force for human development as exemplified by the following quotes:

- 'anyone who cares about the poor should favour the growth-enhancing policies of good rule of law, fiscal discipline, and openness to international trade'. (Dollar and Kraay, 2001)
- 'the new feature of market economics in present day capitalism . . . [is] turbo-capitalism . . . Whoever thinks that the stability of families and communities is important cannot at the same time speak in favour of deregulation and globalization of the economy.' (Luttwak, 1995)

Supporters of current forms of economic globalization can be described as 'globalists'. Globalists support what can neatly be summarized as the Washington Consensus. This set of ideas has, for example, underpinned SAPs, as well as much development aid since the early 1980s.

On the link between globalization and health, globalists would argue that:

- liberalization increases flows of trade and finance;
- trade increases growth, especially in poorer countries;
- growth increases incomes, especially for the poor, so eventually there is a convergence of wealth (i.e. trickle down effect);

- higher incomes mean more resources for governments to spend on health services; and
- higher incomes for the poor means better living conditions and hence improved health status.

These assumed causal links lead to the overall conclusion that globalization is good for health. Globalists argue that all countries need to integrate with the emerging global economy, and where some countries suffer adverse effects, it is because they have not embraced globalization sufficiently.

What evidence supports these policy prescriptions? The work of Dollar and Kraay (2001) is seminal in this debate. They argue that countries that have embraced economic globalization over the past two decades have benefited most. Less globalized countries have suffered negative growth in GDP, while more globalized low income countries have enjoyed growth (over 5%) higher even than high income countries (Figure 6.3).

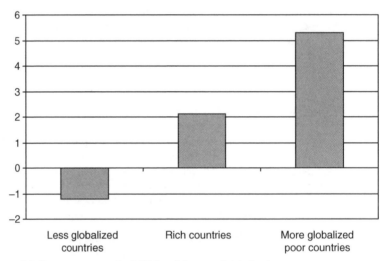

Figure 6.3 Percentage growth of GDP and degree of globalization
Source: Dollar D and Kraay A (2001).

Over the past 40 years, they argue, more globalized countries have enjoyed increasing growth in GDP (Figure 6.4).

Wages are also shown to have grown more in countries that have become more globalized (Figure 6.5). This reflects the relocation of manufacturing and other labour-intensive jobs from high- to low- and middle-income countries (e.g. footwear and clothing, toys, electronics, automobiles). This suggests that workers in more globalized countries are also benefiting from economic growth.

In stark contrast to globalists is the so-called anti-globalization movement, a diverse collection of interest groups that opposes current forms of economic globalization. It is more accurate to describe this group as anti Washington Consensus, rather than globalization per se. They argue that contemporary globalization is:

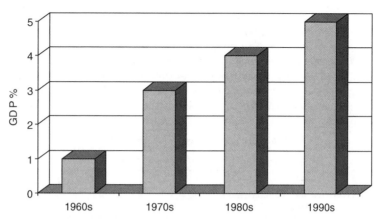

Figure 6.4 Per capita growth for more globalized countries
Source: Dollar and Kraay (2001).

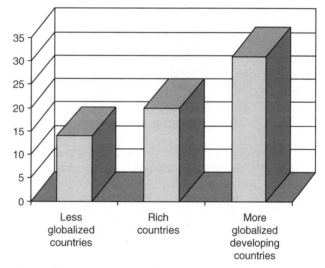

Figure 6.5 Wage growth by degree of globalization
Source: World Bank (2002).

- increasing poverty;
- widening socio-economic inequalities within and between countries;
- creating greater job insecurity;
- weakening workers' rights;
- undermining social welfare and environmental protection; and
- weakening democracy by enabling a global ruling class to act without sufficient transparency and accountability.

Many groups seeking to redirect economic globalization to alleviate poverty, achieve social justice and ensure sustainable growth cite statistical evidence of the adverse impacts of recent trends. One measure is the Gini coefficient which measures inequality within and between countries, and seen to be a truer measure of inequality within countries than GDP per capita. It is estimated that, between the 1950s and 1990s, 48 countries saw a rise in inequality (half the world's population), nine had less inequality, and 16 showed no trend (Table 6.5).

Table 6.5 Trends in inequality (1950s to 1990s)

Trend in inequality	Number of countries	% of world population
Rising	48	47
Falling	9	4
No trend	16	29

Source: Cornia (2001).

There is also concern about the social consequences of the so-called 'race to the bottom'. The greater ease by which capital can flow around the world means TNCs seek the most profitable locations in which to invest. This can mean investing in countries offering relatively cheap sources of inputs (including labour), and favourable tax and regulatory policies. Countries competing to attract foreign direct investment are tempted to relax health and safety regulations for workers, environmental standards and tax rates. For many workers in the global economy, this can mean lower wages and unsafe working conditions.

Shiva (as quoted in Mander, 2000) writes that 'Globalisation of the economy is a new kind of colonialism visited upon poor countries and the poor in rich countries.' This seems supported by the proliferation of 'sweatshops' worldwide as countries seek to increase their global competitiveness by reducing production costs. The working conditions of factories for companies such as Nike, Disney and GAP have attracted public attention in recent years:

- In American Samoa, Vietnamese and Chinese workers have been recruited by an agency to work at a factory making designer clothing for the US department stores, Sears and JC Penney. The workers earn US$200 per month, are given room and board consisting of a bunk in a 36-bed dormitory, and are fed three meagre meals a day. It is reported that pay is routinely withheld, workers regularly beaten, and living conditions squalid. The factories are located in American Samoa because it is a US territory and thus does not attract import duties. The clothing is labelled 'Made in the USA'. Given that the territory is badly in need of investment and employment, and the economy is lightly regulated, investors from South Korea, Taiwan and the Philippines have also begun to set up shop there.
- In China's Guangdong province, young women work 150 hours of overtime each month in garment factories. Sixty per cent do not have a written contract, and 90% have no access to social insurance.
- In Honduras, the government has proposed labour reforms that will permit garment factories to hire up to 30% of their workers on temporary contracts. This is expected to result in job insecurity, loss of paid leave, social security and annual bonus.

The apparent contradiction in data by globalists and its critics can easily confuse. Is globalization resulting in increased growth or reduced incomes? Is the developing world benefiting from economic globalization or becoming ever poorer? With the exception of the most hardened globalists, and most radical anti-globalization activists, what is increasingly clear is that globalization is creating patterns of winners and losers that cut across national borders. There is a need to tease apart aggregated datasets and to determine who are the specific winners and losers across a global economy. Population groups within and across countries need to be considered in terms of variations in total wealth, income distribution, resources, human capital, geography, infrastructure and so on. No one policy, such as full-scale trade liberalization or privatization of state-owned industries, is suitable for all sectors in all countries. This was the approach of SAPs which, while bringing some benefits to some populations, proved harmful for others. Moreover, understanding the health impacts of globalization requires recognition that the playing field is far from level. Economic globalization brings more benefits to those who are educated, have access to the information superhighway, have secure employment, and are relatively mobile. For others, policy measures are needed to remedy these disadvantages.

The work of Milanovic (1999) on household survey data is useful in this respect. He analyses the impacts of trade liberalization on income distribution within rich and poor countries. This means looking not only at rich and poor countries in aggregate, but rich and poor households within different countries. Analysing the impact of openness and FDI as share of country's GDP on relative income of low and high deciles (10%) of population, he found that, in low-income countries, economic globalization tends to benefit the well off. In middle-income countries (e.g. Colombia, Czech Republic, Malaysia), the incomes of the poor and middle-class rise relative to the well off. This is attributed to the availability of basic education which enables more people to participate in the changing economy. He concludes that 'only when at least basic education becomes the norm, can even the poor deciles share benefits of increased labour demand; then inequality falls'.

In summary, the greatest challenge for economic globalization is to improve the current balance sheet of winners and losers. More efforts are needed to identify the most vulnerable, how they are disadvantaged by the changes taking place around us, and the measures needed to enable them to benefit from globalization too. How do we also protect those individuals and population groups that are vulnerable? What social policy measures are needed? How do we protect the environment as economic globalization spreads?

🖉 Activity 6.3

As you read the following article by Richard Feachem (2001), note the economic assumptions that lie behind its key arguments. To what extent do you agree with these arguments?

Globalisation is good for your health, mostly

We live in extraordinary times. Since December 1999 in Seattle, every meeting of the leaders of the World Trade Organisation, the World Bank, the International

Monetary Fund, and the world's richest nations (the G8) has been met by increasingly large and violent demonstrations against global processes that are manifestly beneficial. The protestors comprise such a diverse array of groups and opinions that it is impossible to capture their message in a single phrase (how simple were the anti-Vietnam war protests by comparison). The central theme of the protests is discernible, however, and is something like: 'Increasing global economic and social integration is a conspiracy by the rich and powerful to exploit the poor and underprivileged.'

Beyond this central theme one hears strands that are against capitalism, economic growth, multinational companies, international institutions, and the governments of wealthy countries. Strangely, the protesters are muted or silent in their objection to the corrupt and inefficient governments of some low income countries or to the massive human rights abuses that occur daily in some poorer countries.

The protestors are right about two things. Firstly, poverty is indeed the most pressing moral, political, and economic issue of our time. Secondly, the tide of globalisation can be turned back. However, to reverse that tide would be, in the words of an *Economist* editorial, 'an unparalleled catastrophe for the planet's most desperate people and something that could be achieved only by trampling down individual liberty on a daunting scale.'

Many formal definitions of globalisation have been proposed. I think of it as openness: openness to trade, to ideas, to investment, to people, and to culture. It brings benefits today, as it has for centuries – and it also brings risks and adverse consequences, as it has for centuries.

There are three main flaws in the protesters' positions. Firstly, they overlook a substantial body of rigorous evidence on the economic benefits of globalisation. Secondly, they ignore the wider social and political benefits of globalisation. Thirdly, they lack a counter proposal – if not globalisation, then what?

Economic benefits of globalisation
The evidence that openness to trade and investment is good for economic growth is compelling and goes back several centuries. We can see this effect not only in the multi-country econometric analyses but also in the recent experiences of individual countries. China, India, Uganda, and Vietnam, for example, have all experienced surges in economic growth since liberalising their trade and inward investment policies. Because gross national product per capita correlates so strongly with national health status, we can conclude that, in general, openness to trade improves national health status.

However, evidence on associations between openness and growth among nations does not directly address issues of equity. Recently, it has become common to assert that globalisation has increased inequity both among and within countries. Statements to this effect litter the literature on globalisation and health and are unquestioningly accepted as true in many public health forums. It is necessary to be critical and cautious about such statements. While it will always be possible to show some increasing wealth gaps – especially by comparing very poor countries with very rich countries or by comparing the poorest tenth with the richest tenth within a country – there is strong evidence in the counter direction. For example, globalising developing countries (those which increased trade and reduced import tariffs) have grown much faster than other developing countries. Importantly, they have also grown faster than the wealthy countries in the Organisation for Economic Cooperation and Development (OECD), therefore narrowing the wealth gap between rich and poor countries.

But what of intra-country equity? Again, recent evidence is optimistic. Analysis of 137 countries shows that the incomes of the poorest 20% on average rise and fall in step with national growth or recession. In other words, on average, changes in national wealth are not systematically associated with income distribution. There is, however, considerable individual country variation around this average outcome, and studying the outliers in detail would be fruitful. Why is it that in some countries the poor benefit disproportionately from growth while in others they have been left behind. The answer surely lies in the detail of the economic and social policies in place in those countries at the time that national growth was occurring, and understanding these relationships in detail will help to ensure that the poor always benefit from growth.

It is also important in discussing equity and globalisation to focus on the absolute poverty of nations and of households and not only on poverty relative to the rich. Thus, while some gaps may increase, it may still be the case that poor nations and poor households are getting richer. This is good for them and for their health – even if some nations and households are getting richer and healthier more rapidly.

In summary, globalisation, economic growth, and improvements in health go hand in hand. Economic growth is good for the incomes of the poor, and what is good for the incomes of the poor is good for the health of the poor. Globalisation is a key component of economic growth. Openness to trade and the inflow of capital, technology, and ideas are essential for sustained economic growth.

Social and political benefits of globalisation

For a country to isolate itself from the benefits of globalisation is, in general, to condemn its citizens to unnecessary and protracted poverty and misery. Isolationism also allows unscrupulous and oppressive governments to continue to be unscrupulous and oppressive without fear of condemnation or intervention from the outside. Would the campaigns against corruption and government malpractice be as well informed and as strong as they are in the absence of globalisation and information technology? Would Aung San Suu Kyi still be alive if the rest of the world was not watching her every move? Would genocide in East Timor have been cut short in an unglobalised world? Many very poor people in the world do not have governments that are concerned for their welfare and their interests. Such poor people are given hope by an interconnected world in which information and ideas flow rapidly and protest and action can be mobilised in the face of oppression, corruption, and genocide.

The global movement to improve the rights and prospects of women worldwide, which still has a long way to go, would have nothing like its present moral or practical force in the world in the absence of continuing globalisation. We may lament the tendency for cultural globalisation, although as I travel the world I find that local cultural diversity is alive and well. However, without a trend towards global moral and ethical standards, more Chinese women would still be crippled by foot binding, more African women would still be genitally mutilated, and more Indian women would be killed or beaten in disputes over dowries. Are these advances worth the eyesore of the McDonald's outlet in Hyderabad or a charming market town in rural France? We must each weigh the outcomes.

Technology and its diffusion are another piece of the globalisation story with important implications for health. The pace of technological change is exponential. Ninety per cent of all scientists who have ever lived are alive today. The human genome has been mapped more rapidly than could have been imagined. The explosion of information technology is making it far easier and far cheaper to communicate globally. In 1930 a three minute telephone call from New York to London cost over $300, today it costs 30 cents.

The previous G8 meeting in Okinawa lamented the digital divide. What is more remarkable is the speed at which information technology has reached low income countries and even quite remote areas within those countries. No previous technological revolution, such as steam engines, electricity, or telephones, has diffused so widely and so quickly. Non-governmental organisations in towns in India or Tanzania are now able to connect with like-minded people around the world, perhaps to organise the next anti-globalisation street protests. In terms of connectivity to the internet, Singapore has overtaken the whole of Europe, South Korea does as well as Britain, and middle and large low income countries are increasing their internet connectivity rapidly. Already 0.5% of Indians (five million people) have online access, and this number is set to rise rapidly during the next five years.

The internet itself will have a substantial health impact in low and middle income countries. There are two reasons for this. Firstly, the internet will promote more rapid economic growth than would otherwise have occurred, and this economic growth, in the presence of sound public policy, will promote better incomes and better health for the poor. There are many pathways by which the internet will boost the economy, all of which essentially mean a greater ability for companies in developing countries, especially small ones, to participate in global trade and commerce. Secondly, the communications, data management, and administrative capacity offered by the internet will greatly improve the management and delivery of healthcare services, the surveillance of communicable disease, the response to epidemics, the monitoring of antibiotic resistance, and a host of other important applications in the health sector. We have not yet begun to see the benefits of this application of information technology in most countries.

Alternatives to globalisation

But every silver lining has a cloud. The shift with development from food scarcity to food surplus is accompanied by rising obesity and its associated health consequences. The steady reduction in mortality rates (until HIV infection and AIDS came along) has allowed people to live long enough to develop unpleasant chronic and degenerative diseases, and so with globalisation, a process that has unquestionably brought benefits to many countries, also carries with it risks and negative consequences.

This is not new. Perhaps the most devastating impact of globalisation was the spread of deadly epidemics that accompanied European expansion and colonisation between roughly 1500 and 1800. These epidemics decimated immunologically naïve populations, especially in the Americas and Oceania. Global spread of infection continues today, although (with the notable exception of AIDS) we now have better knowledge and tools with which to ameliorate the consequences.

In addition to the threats from emerging and re-emerging infections that are increased by globalisation, there is the massive debate on global environmental change and its health consequences. I have no doubt that there are grave concerns to be researched and addressed in this area. However, it is noteworthy that the widely held pessimism of the public health community has now been comprehensively challenged.

Conclusions

The protesters derailed the Seattle meeting of the World Trade Organisation and seriously disrupted the G8 summit in Genoa. This despite the fact that matters of vital importance to poor people and to developing countries were being discussed at these meetings. In November in Doha, the World Trade Organisation's 142 member countries will try to launch a new round of global trade negotiations. On the agenda are agricultural tariffs, an area in which the rich countries are notoriously protectionist. Reaching new international agreements on freer trade, particularly in agriculture, is far more important to the lives of the poor than debt relief. Let the health and medical community worldwide give all support to the World Trade Organisation and to the Doha meeting in the name of poverty alleviation and better health for all.

 Feedback

Clearly, the extent to which you agree with the writer's views will depend on the weight you put on different arguments and counter-arguments. Overall, the article contains many of the policy assumptions associated with the Washington Consensus.

Summary

Globalization is most frequently associated with changes emerging from economic globalization which are impacting on societies across the world. The growth and spread of the global economy (trade and finance) is likely to continue apace, creating new opportunities and risks for health. Chapter 7 now considers in greater detail the health implications of trade liberalization under the World Trade Organization.

References

ABN-AMRO Bank. Available at www.abnamro.com. 2005.

Anderson S and Cavanagh J (2000) *Top 200, The Rise of Global Corporate Power*, Washington DC: Institute of Policy Studies. Available at: http://www.ips-dc.org/downloads/Top_200.pdf.

Christian Aid (2002) 'World Social Forum 31 January–5 February 2002'. Available at: http://www.christian-aid.org.uk/wefwsf/wsf.htm.

Cornia GA (2001) 'Globalization and Health: Results and Options,' *Bulletin of the World Health Organization*, 79(9): 834–41.

Dollar D and Kraay A (2001) Growth is Good for the Poor, World Bank Policy Research Department Working Paper No. 2587, Washington DC. Available at: http://www. worldbank.org/research/growth.

Feachem R (2001) 'Globalisation is good for your health . . . mainly, *BMJ*: 323, 504–6.

Longworth R (1998) *Global Squeeze: The Coming Crisis for First-World Nations*. Chicago: Contemporary Books.

Luttwak E (1995) as quoted in Martin and Schuman (1996) *The Global Trap*. London: Pluto Press.

Mander J (2000) 'Corporate Colonialism'. Resurgence, 179. Available at: http://resurgence.gn.apc.org/articles/mander.htm.

Milanovic B (1999) *True World Income Distribution, 1988 and 1993: First Calculations, Based on Household Surveys Alone*, Poverty Working Paper No. 2244, World Bank, Washington DC. http://econ.worldbank.org/files/978_wps2244.pdf.

Scholte JA (2000) 'What is "Global" about Globalization?' In *Globalization, a critical introduction* (Scholte JA, ed.) London: Macmillan: 41–61.

Werner D and Sanders D (1997) *Questioning the Solution: The Politics of Primary Health Care and Child Survival*. Palo Alto: Health Rights.

Williamson J (1990) *Latin American Adjustment: How much has happened?* Washington DC: Institute for International Economics.

World Bank (2002), *Globalization, Growth and Poverty*, World Bank Policy Research Report, Washington DC.

7 The World Trade Organization and public health

Overview

In this chapter you will learn about the World Trade Organization (WTO) and, in particular, the potential implications of multilateral trade agreements for public health. You will cover the history of the international trading system, basic principles underpinning trade law, and the key multilateral trade agreements governing trade today. You will then consider the relevance, in particular, of the Agreement on Trade Related Property Rights (TRIPS) and General Agreement on Services (GATS) for public health.

Learning objectives

After working through this chapter you will be able to:

- describe the origins, structure and functions of the WTO, and the multilateral trade agreements under its management
- recognize the broad ways in which trade issues can be relevant for public health
- understand the basic parameters of the TRIPS and GATS and their potential relevance for public health.

Key terms

Compulsory license The permission given by a government to a third party to use or produce an invention without the consent of the patent holder.

Most favoured nation principle In a trade agreement between two countries, if either party to the treaty grants a favour (usually a tariff reduction) to a third country, the other party to the treaty will be granted the same favour.

Non tariff barrier Barriers to trade that are either quota or quantitative restrictions deliberately designed to protect domestic industries or internal taxes, administrative requirements, health and sanitary regulations and government procurement policies that are not necessarily intended to restrict trade.

Parallel import The importation of a product without the approval of the owner of patent or trademark or copyright.

Tariff A tax levied against an imported good or service.

A brief history of the world trading system

Trade between different societies has occurred throughout history, with rules governing trade relations becoming more formalized as societies have developed. Complex systems of *tariffs* evolved whereby trading parties may impose taxes on imports to encourage or discourage the trade of certain goods. During the eighteenth century, principles were developed among leading trading nations to facilitate the crossborder movement of goods. Perhaps the most important is the *most favoured nation* (MFN) principle which states that, in a trade agreement between two countries, if either party to the treaty grants a favour (usually a tariff reduction) to a third country, the other party to the treaty will be granted the same favour. The First World War (1914–19), and events thereafter, led to a weakening of the application of this principle. This resulted in the escalating and punitive application of tariffs by many governments and a major depression in the world economy.

Following the Second World War, efforts were made to create a new system of international trade that would prevent 'tit for tat' protectionism from threatening peace and stability again. The original plan was to create a permanent International Trade Organization (ITO) as agreed in Havana, Cuba in 1948. The ITO would be an equal ranking institution to the World Bank and International Monetary Fund (see Chapter 6). Its work would be based around a General Agreement on Trade and Tariffs (GATT), signed by 23 states in 1947, as part of a more stable world economy. In the end, the ITO was not created when the US government declined to ratify its charter and the GATT, by default, became the only multilateral agreement governing world trade.

The institutional framework of GATT became the driving force behind trade liberalization over the next 50 years. It served as the forum for negotiating reductions in tariffs through a series of 'trade rounds' held between 1947 and 1994. Table 7.1 lists these trade rounds, the number of countries participating, and trade concessions achieved. Notable is the growth in number of countries involved, the broadened scope of subjects under negotiation and, not unrelated, length of time taken for rounds to conclude.

Table 7.1 Trade rounds held under the GATT from 1947–1994

Trade round	No. of countries participating	Subject of negotiations
Geneva Round (1947)	23 countries	Concessions on 43 tariff lines
Annency Round (1949)	29 countries	Modest reductions
Torquay Round (1950–51)	32 countries	8,700 concessions
Geneva Round (1955–56)	33 countries	Modest reductions
Dillon Round (1960–61)	39 countries	Formation of EEC 4,400 concessions
Kennedy Round (1963–67)	74 countries	Anti-dumping, customs valuation, preferential treatment to LDCs
Toyko Round (1973–79)	99 countries	1/3 tariff reduction by DCs, codes of conduct on NTBs
Uruguay Round (1986–94)	124 countries	1/3 tariff reduction by DCs, agriculture, clothing, GATS, TRIPS, WTO created

Since 1945, international trade has rapidly increased in scale and scope. A wave of trade liberalization occurred from the 1970s to mid-1990s. Throughout this period, there was an increase in the signing of bilateral (between two countries) and regional (within geographical region) trade agreements. The most sought after bilateral trade partner was the US given the size of its import market. Regional agreements included the North American Free Trade Agreement (NAFTA), Asian Free Trade Agreement (AFTA), Europe Union (EU) and Andean Common Market (ANCOM). These agreements and many more contributed to a reduction in tariffs (Figure 7.1) which fell on average from around 40% in 1940 to 4% in 1995. Consequently, crossborder trade has intensified measured by the ratio of world trade to world output (or national trade to GDP minus government expenditure). There has also been an increase in the number of countries/territories involved in the international trading system.

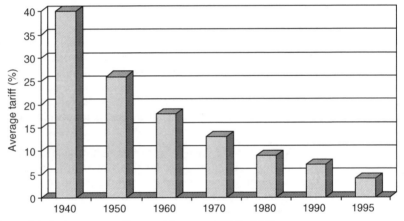

Figure 7.1 Reduction in tariffs in world economy (1940–1995)

Source: Dicken (1996).

The creation of the World Trade Organization

The most significant trade round of GATT was the Uruguay Round which lasted almost eight years (1986–94). Its conclusion led to the replacement of the GATT with the World Trade Organization (WTO) in 1995. As well as being a permanent institution, trade rules under the WTO expanded beyond trade in goods to cover services and intellectual property rights. Its stated functions are to:

- serve as a forum for trade negotiations, monitoring national trade policies and settling trade disputes;
- carry out day-to-day administration of trade agreements under its jurisdiction;
- assist member states in implementing trade agreements; and
- oversee special arrangements for low-income countries in their compliance with trade agreements.

The latter, however, does not mean that WTO is a funding body. Indeed, it has no mandate to finance development projects. Rather, the organization provides special and preferential treatment to low-income countries in the form of exemptions from certain obligations or reciprocity, longer transition periods and technical assistance. For example, it offers training to officials in understanding the trading system, administration of agreements, and taking effective part in trade negotiations.

In October 2004 there were 148 member states of the WTO. Together they account for more than 90% of world trade. It is notable that this figure excludes what is believed to be a huge 'informal' or parallel economy including the global trade in illicit drugs, counterfeit goods, and even people trafficking, all of which have health-related consequences. Membership in the WTO is by no means automatic, but must be negotiated with existing member states. After a membership application is submitted, a working party is set up by the General Council (see below) which, while open to all member states, usually consists of those countries with an interest in the applicant country's trade regime. The applicant government presents a memorandum covering all aspects of its trade and legal regime to the working party. At the same time, the applicant government engages in bilateral negotiations with interested working party members on concessions and commitments on market access for goods and services. The results of these bilateral negotiations are consolidated into a document which is part of the final 'accession package'. The entire process can take several years, with China's accession in 2001 taking 14 years of negotiation. Importantly, with so many countries now members, there is pressure to join for any country seeking to trade.

The WTO is based in Geneva with 500 staff headed by a Director-General (Figure 7.2). Its top decision-making body is the Ministerial Conference which brings together leading trade officials of member states at least once every two years. The General Council meets several times a year in Geneva and is attended by ambassadors, representatives of those countries with permanent trade delegations in Geneva, or officials from member states (which may include health experts). The General Council also meets as the Trade Policy Review Body and the Dispute Settlement Body (DSB). The annual budget of the WTO is around US$100 million.

The overall principles underpinning the world trading system under the WTO are:

- most favoured nation treatment;
- trade without discrimination;
- use of tariffs to ensure predictable and increased access to markets;
- promotion of fair competition;
- encouragement of development and economic reform; and
- transparency.

These principles are set out in the GATT (for goods), and the General Agreement on Trade in Services (for services). Additional agreements deal with the special requirements of specific sectors or issues. Some have detailed and lengthy schedules (or lists) of commitments made by individual countries. In services, for example, the commitments state how much access a foreign service provider is allowed for a specific sector.

One important innovation of the WTO is the creation of a new procedure for settling trade disputes. Formal dispute settlement is an option of last resort.

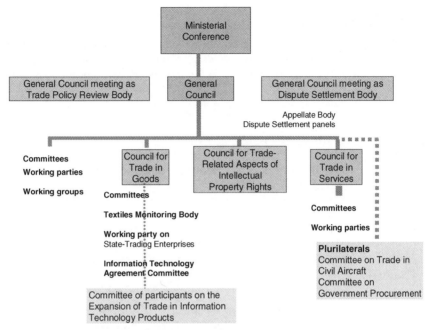

Figure 7.2 Structure of the World Trade Organization
Source: WHO (2002).

Nevertheless, if two or more WTO members have a dispute over a trade measure and cannot resolve it between themselves (or in other fora), they have the right to bring the dispute to the Dispute Settlement Body (DSB) of the WTO (the General Council in another guise). A dispute can only be brought between member states, and only about alleged failures to comply with WTO agreements or commitments. Companies, organizations or private individuals cannot complain directly to the WTO, but can do so through a member state. When a dispute is lodged, a panel of experts is established by the DSB to consider the case. The WTO then has the sole authority to accept or reject panels' findings or the results of an appeal. It monitors implementation of rulings and recommendations from panels and the Appellate Body. It also has the power to authorize compensation or suspension of concessions if a country fails to comply with a ruling.

✏ **Activity 7.1**

In your home can you find ten items that have been imported from other countries? How many items can you find imported from different continents? Is there one country or region where most of your imported goods come from?

Feedback

> It should not be difficult to find imported goods in your home. Most are likely to come from countries or regions that have special trading relationships with your home country, or from countries that lead the world in manufacturing such as China and the US.

Protection of trade versus public health

While historical precedent and powerful vested interests have given substantial weight to international trade law, there have been efforts to balance its application with other policy objectives including public health. A notable exception to the MFN principle is that a member state may restrict trade on goods and/or services when necessary to protect the health of humans, animals and plants on the condition that either the restriction is applied in a non-discriminatory way or the restriction is based on recognized scientific evidence (Article XX, GATT). Article XVI of the General Agreement on Trade in Services (see below) authorizes similar restriction on services and service suppliers.

The first requirement suggests that, if the intention is to protect the consumer, it should not matter where the health risk originates. This does not mean that if a government allows imports of a particular product from one country, it must allow imports of the same product from all countries. For example, the same fish product might be allowed in from one country but banned from another because it is contaminated with cholera. The same requirement must apply to all countries, but will affect them differently depending on the health status of their product.

The second requirement means that a trade restriction cannot be a disguised form of protectionism. Measures taken to restrict trade must be no more than is necessary. There is no requirement under Article XX of GATT to quantify the risk to human life or health. To determine whether a restrictive measure is necessary requires a weighing and balancing of factors which include:

- the importance of the interests protected by the measure;
- the efficacy of such measure in pursuing the policies; and
- the impact of the law or regulation on imports or exports.

There are examples of disputes arising from trade restrictions in an effort to protect public health. A WTO member state can challenge the imposition of such measures through the Dispute Settlement Body (described above) if it feels there are unfair trade practices at play. Evidence sustaining the restrictive measure must be of recognized scientific standards, and the use of the so-called 'precautionary principle' to avert potential versus proven risk/harm to health (as you will see in Chapter 10), as a basis for limiting trade, remains subject to dispute. A good example is food imports. A country may decide, for instance, to restrict an imported fruit because of what it deems an unacceptable level of pesticide presence. This is a perfectly legitimate public health concern and, if applied in a non-discriminatory way (all member states treated the same) and based on scientific principles (research shows this to be a risk), it is a justifiable trade barrier under WTO rules. A dispute can arise, however, where the scientific evidence is unclear or contentious. The dispute between the European Community and US government over the import of hormone-treated beef into EC member states arose from disagreement over the scientific evidence on the true risk. The dispute arose in 1988 when the EC prohibited the use of hormonal substances for animal growth promotion including 17β oestradiol, testosterone, progesterone, zeranol, trenbolone acetate and melengestrol acetate (MGA). The ban applies without discrimination internally and to all imports from third countries from 1 January 1989. Third countries wishing to export bovine meat and meat products to the European Community had to either have equivalent legislation or to operate a hormone-free cattle programme. Some 90% of US cattle producers routinely use hormones to make cattle grow faster and bigger. After the ban was imposed, the US exported only hormone-free beef to the EU, losing an estimated US$500 million annually. A series of trade sanctions have been imposed by the US and Canada in response. The EU prohibition has been maintained despite two rulings that it does not comply with WTO commitments, and the EU has sought to reopen the issue at the DBS/WTO based on new evidence. The WTO ruling, that the EU had to remove the import ban, led to criticisms of the expertise used to assess the risk, and the scope permitting application of the precautionary principle. In contrast, a dispute between the European Community and Canadian government over the banning in 1997 of imported asbestos by the French government resulted in an upholding of the import ban by the WTO in 2000 on the grounds of protecting public health (WTO, 2001). The two cases demonstrate that, while the WTO provides scope to protect public health, this is strongly dependent on the availability of 'clear' scientific evidence.

A future area of dispute is likely to be trade in goods and services that are inherently harmful to health. Tobacco products are perhaps the best example but one might also include the international arms trade and toxic waste. According to economic theory, free trade generally leads to increased competition, improved efficiency and lower prices. All of these factors, in turn, lead to increased production and consumption of the traded product. This is assumed to be beneficial when concerned with 'goods'. However, public health advocates argue that tobacco products should be considered 'bads', with increased production and consumption leading to greater harm in the form of greater death and disease. Evidence showing that trade liberalization of tobacco products has led to an increase in consumption, and thus adverse health impact, in low-income countries (Bettcher et al., 2000). The tobacco industry has actively lobbied in bilateral, regional and multilateral trade forums for its products to be treated like any other good. Public health advocates argue that tobacco should be treated differently, allowing countries to restrict its trade. This is likely to be an important area of tension between trade and health in forthcoming trade negotiations on the agriculture sector.

✏ **Activity 7.2**

Make a list of goods and services that you think might pose a direct risk to public health if traded from one country to another. Describe how such a risk might emerge.

Feedback

Some examples of goods include tobacco products, contaminated foodstuffs, toxic chemicals and military weapons. Examples of potentially risky services are unregulated health services, such as alternative therapies, or inappropriate advertising messages. Think about potential health risks that may arise from the time a good or service arrives into the country, to their purchase and use by the end consumer.

Agreement on Trade Related Intellectual Property Rights (TRIPS) and access to medicines

A new feature of the WTO, not present under GATT, is the Agreement on Trade Related Aspects of Intellectual Property Rights (TRIPS) adopted at the end of the Uruguay Round in 1995. The agreement sets out minimum standards for protecting and enforcing nearly all forms of intellectual property rights (i.e. patents, trademarks and copyright) for member states, with standards derived from legislation in industrialized countries. All member states must comply with these standards, where necessary modifying their national legislation. Importantly, the agreement (Article 8) explicitly acknowledges that, in framing national laws, members 'may . . . adopt measures necessary to protect public health and nutrition, and to promote the public interest.'

In an important departure from previous conventions, pharmaceutical products are accorded full intellectual property rights (IPR) under TRIPS. Pharmaceutical companies are granted the legal means, as patent owners of new drug products, to prevent others from making, using or selling the new invention for a limited period of time. The TRIPS agreement specifies that patents must be available for all discoveries which 'are new, involve an inventive step and are capable of industrial application' (Article 27). Patent protection can thus be obtained for new drug products that enable the patent holder to have exclusive rights to produce and sell the product. Pharmaceutical companies argue that such rights, and the consequent ability to charge a higher price for a drug under patent, is necessary to recoup the many millions of dollars spent to research and develop the drug, and bring it to market. Without the prospect of earning such prices, the incentive to invest in research and development (R&D) would be seriously undermined (WTO, 2003). As stated by Sidney Taurel (2003), CEO of Eli Lilly, the 'whole process of pharmaceutical innovation is made possible – viable – by two important features of our economic system: one is market-based pricing . . . the other is intellectual property protection.'

Within the public health community, TRIPS raises concerns about access to medicines. For drugs unprotected by patent rights, because such rights are not granted, asserted or have expired, other producers can manufacture generic versions that can be sold more competitively. This leads to lower drug prices for consumers, especially important for low-income countries. However, for drugs under patent protection, producers are allowed to charge higher prices. Where a drug is needed for an important public health condition, the high cost of patented drugs becomes a particularly acute issue (WHO, 2001). This tension between the economics of drug development and marketing, and the need to protect public health, came to a head in 2001 when the South African government sought an amendment to the South African Medicines and Related Substances Control Amendment Act that would allow the import and use of cheaper generic versions of prescription drugs. This amendment was sought to allow the country to import cheaper anti-retroviral (ARVs) for help tackle the country's serious HIV/AIDS problem. The key clause stated that the government could find and 'parallel import' the cheapest drug available, and grant 'compulsory licensing' to other companies allowing them to make copies of patented drugs without the patent holder's permission. It was argued that the rapidly rising prevalence of HIV/AIDS in the country was a public health emergency. Thirty-nine pharmaceutical companies, including GlaxoSmithKline, Merck and Roche, did not agree and launched a legal action in 1998 to protect their patents.

The case was eventually dropped by the drug companies in April 2001 following campaigning by non-governmental organizations such as Health Action International and Medicin sans Frontières (MSF). Despite seeing the South African action as a test case to prevent other countries, such as Brazil and India, from following suit, the companies faced unexpected negative publicity and strong criticism. The clear need to further clarify the terms of the TRIPS agreement was thus recognized. In 2001, at the Ministerial Conference of the WTO held in Doha, Qatar, a Declaration on TRIPS and Public Health was agreed (known as the Doha Declaration) recognizing the right of WTO members to 'protect public health and, in particular, to promote access to medicines for all'. In addition, Paragraph 6 of the Doha Declaration instructed the TRIPS Council to address how WTO members with insufficient manufacturing capacities in pharmaceuticals can make effective use of compulsory licensing. While these countries may issue compulsory licences to import generic versions of patent-protected medicines, TRIPS rules impose constraints on the abilities of countries to authorize exports of such products. Paragraph 6 promised a solution to the export problem caused by these constraints and a further agreement to address this problem was reached in August 2003 (Correa, 2004).

General Agreement on Trade in Services (GATS) and trade in health services

In the past, most services were not considered to be tradeable across borders. Much has changed to alter the tradability of services, including health services. Advances in communications technology, including the rise of e-commerce, and regulatory changes have made it easier to deliver services across borders. In many countries, changes in government policy have left greater room for the private sector – domestic as well as foreign – to provide services. Partly as a result of this, services have become the fastest-growing segment of the world economy, providing more than 60% of global output and employment. Such changes led governments to call for the inclusion of services in trade negotiations. The result was the General Agreement on Trade in Services (GATS) agreed at the end of the Uruguay Round.

GATS defines four modes of service delivery:

- **Mode 1** – Cross-border supply, e.g. provision of diagnosis or treatment planning services in country A by suppliers in country B, via telecommunications ('telemedicine');

- **Mode 2** – Consumption abroad, e.g. movement of patients from country A to country B for treatment;
- **Mode 3** – Commercial presence, e.g. establishment of or investment in hospitals in country A whose owners are from country B; and
- **Mode 4** – Presence of natural persons, e.g. service provision in country A by health professionals who have temporarily left country B to provide services in A.

In relation to trade in health services, there has generally been growth of almost all of these modes and little evidence so far that this is related to GATS (Smith, 2004). Some modes of trade in health services, such as the cross-border (Mode 1) supply of nursing services, are unlikely to be practical. However, other services, such as processing of medical claims processing or transcribing medical records, can be supplied on a cross-border basis. Medical transcription services are a small but fast-growing industry in India. Indian companies transcribe medical records and send the information back to American health facilities via direct satellite link. Consumption of health services abroad (Mode 2) is thought to be growing, with several countries seeing 'health tourism' as an economic development opportunity. Bangkok and Singapore are drawing health consumers from the entire Asian region, for specialized services unavailable in less-developed countries, and in 'health tourism' packages for people from industrialized countries. These countries aim to provide complex tertiary services at lower cost, bundle health services and then market them to foreign patients, or provide services to returning expatriates. Foreign investment in health services or 'commercial presence' (Mode 3) seeks to improve the quality of commercially available health services for those who can afford them, particularly when accompanied by new technology and know-how. This might take the form of investment in a modern hospital or health insurance management practices. By mid-1999 US health insurers had enrolled over 5 million members in Latin America. Chilean and Colombian private health insurance plans are rapidly entering foreign markets (*The Economist*, 8 May 1999). Presence of natural persons (Mode 4), the least significant in total trade flows, is the most visible of the four modes. The migration of health professionals from less developed to more developed countries is the most prominent example. Bangladesh, India, Pakistan and the Philippines, among others, are the source of large numbers of 'exported' health professionals.

GATS takes a gradual approach to trade liberalization. So far the liberalizing effects of GATS on the trade in health services have remained limited. Most WTO members have made relatively few market access commitments that go beyond existing levels. Table 7.2 shows the number of countries that have made such

Table 7.2 Patterns of commitments on health services by WTO member states

	Total number of WTO members (July 2001)	Developing and transitional economies
Medical and dental services	54	36
Nurses, midwives, physiotherapists	29	12
Hospital services	44	29
Other human health services (ambulances, etc)	17	15

Source: WHO 2002.

commitments under GATS. Signatories were allowed to register exceptions to the MFN obligation when GATS came into effect in 1995. Some 400 exemptions were requested. In principle, exemptions should not last more than 10 years, but they will be subject to further negotiation.

Certain principles, called general or unconditional obligations, apply to all WTO members when engaging in trade in all service sectors. These include transparency and notification, exceptions for services supplied in the exercise of government authority, and general exceptions for public order and protection of the health of people, animals or plants. In addition, the MFN principle requires that members treat equally services and suppliers from all WTO members. If a country permits trade in services in a sector, then all suppliers from other member countries must be permitted market access on equal terms. If no trade is permitted in a particular sector, the prohibition must apply equally to suppliers from all countries.

Some provisions under the GATS raise concerns about their applicability to public health services and social health insurance. First, it remains to be seen to what extent government services are excluded (Article I.3). In most countries, public sector health providers coexist with private health providers. Does this make them 'competitive' if they serve similar patients and provide similar services – thus denying exemption to the publicly provided services? If public sector services charge user fees, does that make them commercial? Under current definitions, the answers are not clear. For example, do co-payments or user fees render public services commercial? Under which conditions do public and private providers compete?

Second, what is the scope of the general exception for health (Article XIV)? The general health exception 'for measures *necessary* to protect human. . . . life or health' suggests that national health insurance laws or programmes, because they are designed to protect human health, could be exempt from GATS requirements, as long as they do not discriminate among trading partners. However, WTO case law indicates that this would be subject to strict tests regarding what is 'necessary' to protect health. Providing health coverage through mandatory social health insurance could be regarded as incidental to health protection, rather than essential to allow access to life-saving services. Thus, it remains unclear whether all public health measures are subject to 'necessary' or 'least-trade restrictive' tests.

Finally, there are limitations in the existing data on trade in services which does not disaggregate data by sector. Health services do not appear, except for health-related travel for a few countries. Some industrialized countries that do collect such data mask the information in publications to protect private businesses' confidentiality. Many developing countries lack data collection systems, so data is roughly estimated. It is therefore difficult to discern trends in such trade, and the extent to which GATS has or will impact on them. There remains no global picture of health services trade, only anecdotes and case studies. There is a need for better data to track scale and direction of health services trade over time. This would serve to establish the basis for trade liberalization decisions; and to track changes that result from trade liberalization (Drager and Fidler, 2004).

Activity 7.3

Imagine that you needed a specialized operation but the procedure was not available in your own country. Draw up a list of some of the practical considerations you might need to take into account in seeking this treatment abroad.

 Feedback

You may wish to think about how to find a qualified practitioner, whether language would pose a barrier, how the service would be paid for, and what recourse you would have if the operation was performed incorrectly.

Summary

You have learnt how the WTO is one of the institutional pillars of economic globalization. The various multilateral trade agreements under its jurisdiction influence both the broad determinants of health, as well as the nature of health services and financing, in all countries.

References

Bettcher D, Yach D and Guindon E (2000) 'Global trade and health: key linkages and future challenges'. *Bulletin of the World Health Organization*, 78(4): 521–34.

Correa C (2004) Implementation of the WTO General Council Decision on Para 6 of the Doha Declaration on the TRIPS Agreement and Public Health'. *EDM Series No. 16*, World Health Organization, Geneva.

Dicken P (1996) *Global Shift*. London: Paul Chapman.

Drager N and Fidler D (2004) 'GATS and Health Related Services, Managing Liberalization of Trade in Services From a Health Policy Perspective'. *Trade and Health Notes*, World Health Organization, Geneva, February.

The Economist (1999) 'The Americas shift to private health care', 8 May: 27–9.

Smith R (2004) 'Foreign direct investment and trade in health services: A review of the literature'. *Social Science and Medicine*, 59: 2313–23.

Taurel S (2003) 'Where Drugs Come From – The Facts of Life About Pharmaceutical Innovation'. *Speech to Hudson Institute Forum, National Press Club*. Washington DC, 4 November. Available at: www.ifpma.org/News/SpeechDetail.aspx?nID=498.

WHO (2001) 'Globalization, TRIPS and access to pharmaceuticals'. *WHO Policy Perspectives on Medicines*, No. 3, Geneva, March.

WHO Training Course, 'Public Health Implications of the WTO Multilateral Trade Agreements,' WHO, Geneva, 2002.

WTO (2001) 'European Communities – Measures affecting asbestos and asbestos-containing products'. *Report of the Appellate Body*, 12 March. Available at: www.wto.org.

WTO (2003) 'TRIPS and pharmaceutical patents'. *Fact Sheet*, Geneva, September.

8 The globalization of the pharmaceutical industry

Overview

In this chapter you will examine the structure of the pharmaceutical industry, its consolidation over recent decades, and the particular importance of US companies and the US market in this process. You will consider patented drugs and market bestsellers, research and development (R&D), and the role played by generic drugs. You will then examine the power of the industry, the bodies that regulate it, and the adequacy of the drug approval process. Finally, you will consider the extent to which the industry is globalizing and the consequences of this in relation to globalization.

Learning objectives

After working through this chapter, you should be able to:

- **describe the changing structure of the pharmaceutical industry**
- **consider the relative importance of patented and generic drugs**
- **understand the pharmaceutical industry's sources of power**
- **understand the work of the agencies regulating the activities of the industry, particularly product approval**
- **consider the extent to which the pharmaceutical industry is globalizing and the resultant consequences.**

Key terms

Drug approval agencies National and international bodies that must approve the safety and efficacy of a drug before it can be used.

Generic drug A copy of a medicine produced once its patent protection expires and usually sold under its chemical rather than brand name.

Medicalization The tendency for a range of problems to be defered as medical and therefore at subject to the licence and control of medicine.

Patent A formal licence that an invention cannot be copied in the jurisdiction for which it is applied.

Regulatory capture The process by which an independent regulatory agency takes on the values and interests of the group whose activities it regulates.

How is the pharmaceutical industry structured?

The pharmaceutical industry is a major industry in the world economy whose worldwide sales amounted to US$466 billion in 2003, more than the gross national product of many low-income countries. The market is dominated by a small number of large companies with head offices in the US or Europe. In 1992 the top ten companies accounted for roughly one-third of world revenue (Tarabusi and Vickery, 1998). By 2002, after a period of consolidation, this share increased to nearly one-half. The top ten ranked by sales revenue in 2004 is given in Table 8.1.

Table 8.1 Leading pharmaceutical companies by world sales value (July 2004)*

Company	Rank	Head office
Pfizer	1	US
GlaxoSmithKline	2	Britain
Merck & Co.	3	US
AstraZeneca	4	Britain
Novartis	5	Switzerland
Johnson & Johnson	6	US
Bristol-Myers Squibb	7	US
Aventis	8	France
Wyeth	9	US
Hoffman-La Roche	10	Switzerland

* rankings based on pharmacy purchases.
Source: IMS Health (2004d).

Many of the top ten companies are the result of mergers and acquisitions, often between companies based in different countries. For instance, the US company Pfizer, with sales of US$45.2 billion in 2003, achieved its position as market leader after acquiring Warner-Lambert in 2000 and Pharmacia in 2003. Pharmacia has European origins, created by a merger between KabiVitrum of Sweden and the Italian company Carlo Erba in 1993. Aventis was the product of a merger between the German, Hoechst, and the French, Rhone-Poulenc, also in 1999. And industry consolidation continues. The French company Aventis, ranked eighth, was bought in 2004 by another French company, Sanofi-Synthelabo, ranked sixteenth. This merger is likely to push Sanofi-Aventis to third place, and the share of world revenues of the top ten to over 50% (IMS Health, 2004a). The dominance of US companies is unsurprising given that the US and Canada account for nearly half of world pharmaceutical revenues (Table 8.2).

Leading pharmaceutical companies are among the most profitable in the world. For instance, between 1995 and 2002 pharmaceutical companies topped the list of the most profitable companies in the US. In 2003 the industry dropped to third in profitability, overtaken by mining and crude-oil production and banking, as key products lost patent protection. Nonetheless, drug companies remained three times as profitable (14.3%) as the median for the leading 500 companies (4.6%) in the US (Kaiser Family Foundation, 2004).

The profits of leading companies come largely from the sale of patented drugs. A patent is a governmental grant of ownership over an innovation or idea (known as an intellectual property right). A patent can be claimed if an invention is new,

Table 8.2 World pharmaceutical sales revenue (prescription and over-the-counter sales) by region, 2003

World market	Sales 2003 ($bn)	%	% Growth over year
North America	229.5	49	+11
European Union	115.4	25	+8
Rest of Europe	14.3	3	+14
Japan	52.4	11	+3
Asia, Africa and Australia	37.3	8	+12
Latin America	17.4	4	+6
Total	466.3	100	+9

Source: IMS Health (2004a, b, c, d)

involves an 'inventive step' and is capable of industrial application. The standard length of a patent is 20 years, although there are various means for extending this period, for instance, by making small changes to a product or process. A drug company may seek a patent once a new substance with therapeutic potential is identified in order to secure exclusive rights over its production and commercial use. This allows the company to set a (higher) price by virtue of this exclusivity. Since securing approval for a drug can be a slow process, in practice, the commercial patent life will be considerably less than 20 years (perhaps only half). Nor is this period necessarily free from competition since other companies may seek to produce similar products that are sufficiently different to secure their own patents. Such 'me-too' drugs are common within the industry. For instance, five of the top ten companies currently produce their own cholesterol-lowering statin.

Along with patent protection, substances with their own chemical names are usually given simpler 'brand names' as a way of helping to secure a clear identity in the market and improve sales. These are protected by means of registered trademarks. Registering a name as a trademark allows its use for a finite period, with the possibility of extensions. Brand names are important for sales since they help to differentiate what may be chemically quite similar drugs.

The most successful patented drugs change quite rapidly as new products come onto the market and existing drugs lose protection. The bestsellers by revenue in 2003 are shown in Table 8.3. Two cholesterol-lowering statins headed the bestseller list, and drugs for chronic problems requiring long-term medication, such as ulcers, asthma, depression and high cholesterol, were dominant. These 'blockbusters' were crucial to global sales, with the top ten accounting for just over one-tenth of world revenue.

Innovation, research and development, and biotechnology

Patent protection, which permits a higher price to be charged for a drug, is typically justified by the industry in terms of the high cost of research and development (R&D) needed for product innovation. Leading companies spend around 15% and 16% of revenue on R&D. Whether the cost fully justifies the high prices for patented drugs remains a matter of debate. Certainly the cost of bringing drugs involving new medical entities (NMEs) onto the market can be high, estimated by

Table 8.3 Leading pharmaceutical products in 2003

Product	Treatment indication	Company	FDA approval	2003 sales US$billion	% sales growth
Lipitor® (atorvastatin)	High cholesterol	Pfizer	1996	10.3	14
Zocor® (simvastatin)	High cholesterol	Merck & Co	1991	6.1	−4
Zyprexa® (olanzapine)	Psychosis	Eli Lilly	1996	4.8	13
Norvasc® (amlodipine besylate)	High blood pressure/ angina	Pfizer	1992	4.5	7
Erypo/Eprex/Procrit® (epoetin alfa)	Anaemia	Johnson & Johnson subsidiaries	1999	4.0	13
Ogastro/Prevacid® (lansoprazole)	Ulcers/stomach acid	Abbott Labs/ TAP pharmaceuticals	1995	4.0	10
Nexium® (esomeprazole magnesium)	Heartburn/ stomach acid	AstraZeneca	2001	3.8	62
Plavix® (clopidogrel bisulphate)	Prevention of stroke/heart attacks	Bristol Myers Squibb/Sanofi	1997	3.7	40
Seretide/Advair Diskus® (fluticasone proprionate (corticosteroid)+ salmeterol)	Asthma	GlaxoSmithKline	2000	3.7	40
Zoloft® (sertraline hydrochloride) (SSRI)	Depression	Pfizer	1991	3.4	11
Total				**48.3**	**10.9**

Source: IMS Health (2004f).

the industry at around US$800 million per drug. However, many new drugs are similar to those already on the market and, in these cases, the development costs are lower. One study showed that only 35% of applications to the US Food and Drug Administration (FDA) between 1989 and 2000 related to NMEs (NIHCM, 2002). Moreover pharmaceutical R&D may build on basic research, often funded from the public purse, rather than by the companies themselves.

Increasingly crucial R&D work is also being done by smaller biotechnology companies which, when a product with market potential is identified, may license the discovery to a major pharmaceutical company with the resources and expertise to secure regulatory approval and mount a successful market launch. While many biotechnology companies are located in the US and Europe, a growing number are found in countries like Brazil, Argentina and India. Some are independent; some are being taken over by pharmaceutical companies seeking to gain from their innovative research. For example the British biotechnology company, Celltech, which in 2003 had acquired another biotechnology company, Oxford GlycoSciences, was then taken over by the Belgium pharmaceutical and specialist chemical company UCB in July 2004.

The emerging importance of the biotechnology sector is demonstrated by the proportion (35%) of its products among the NMEs submitted for approval in 2001 (IMS Health, 2004b). Biotechnology products are beginning to emerge among the bestsellers. Eprex®, a drug to treat anaemia, was fifth in the top ten for 2003. Overall the biotechnology market was worth almost US$37 billion in 2003. Currently the biotechnology industry is more concentrated than the pharmaceutical industry, with the top ten companies accounting for 84%. But this concentration could change as new smaller companies develop products with market potential.

Generic pharmaceuticals

Once a drug is out of patent, *generic* versions can legally be produced. The term generic refers either to products or processes that are out of patent, or those that do not have a trademark. Commonly it refers to medicines produced once a patent expires, sold under their chemical rather than brand name, given that trademarks can be protected for longer than patents. For instance, when the patent for Prozac® ended, generic versions began to be sold under the chemical name fluoxetine because Eli Lilly retained the brand name as a registered trademark. While generating less revenue than patented drugs, generics represent a major source of sales volume. For instance, in the US, where revenue from patented drugs is highest, around 45% of prescriptions were dispensed generically in 2001 (IMS Health, 2002).

Generally the production of generic medicines has been less attractive to leading companies than patented drugs since they are less profitable. Consequently, in the US and Europe it has been largely left to specialist companies to produce generic drugs. However, the importance of such companies is growing. In 2003 six generic companies were among the top ten fastest growing pharmaceutical companies globally (IMS Health, 2004c). Some leading pharmaceutical companies are beginning to show more interest in generics. For instance, Novartis has acquired several European generic companies in recent years.

Companies producing generic drugs are located in a number of non-western countries and are more widely distributed globally than those producing patented drugs. Japan is a major market for pharmaceuticals with 11% of world sales revenue. The Japanese industry has been relatively fragmented, with over 1,000 companies, but there are signs of consolidation. Some Japanese companies operate overseas and exports are increasing, but overall Japan is a net importer of pharmaceuticals with foreign companies accounting for around one-third of prescribed drugs. China's industry has also been fragmented with over 6,000 pharmaceutical manufacturers, many of which record losses. However, 60 companies account for 33% of the revenues. About 40% of companies are engaged in joint ventures with foreign companies – in part as a way of circumventing China's strict import regulations. China, however, is currently a net exporter of pharmaceuticals, mostly to non-western countries. Pharmaceutical companies in India have been relatively successful, with some exporting to industrialized markets. These include Ranbaxy, the largest pharmaceutical company in India, and Dr Reddy's Laboratories. Ranbaxy had nearly 5% of the Indian market in 2003, and global sales of US$972 million in 2003. It manufactures in seven countries and spends 6% of revenue on R&D.

Generic drug manufacturers have usually developed to supply drugs to domestic markets, including copies of drugs patented elsewhere. Since the mid-1990s, there have been efforts, notably through the World Trade Organization (WTO), to require all countries to adopt levels of patent protection granted in western countries. This is having some effect, with non-western companies increasingly concentrating on producing only generic drugs, but some of the largest are seeking to develop new drugs or processes that can be patented.

 Activity 8.1

Look at the business section of a major national newspaper over a two-week period. Collect any stories about pharmaceuticals or pharmaceutical companies. What can you observe about the companies or products covered?

 Feedback

You might find that many of the companies are, or are affiliated with, the world's leading companies described in this chapter. If trends in ownership, sales, profits or market growth are discussed, you may wish to think about such trends in relation to the global restructuring of the industry towards larger companies with worldwide reach.

How powerful is the pharmaceutical industry?

Light's (1995) framework concerning countervailing powers is useful when assessing the power of the pharmaceutical industry. Countervailing powers are powers that stand in dynamic relation to one another so that, if one power becomes dominant, it is likely to elicit responses from others to redress this imbalance. Focusing on health care services, Light distinguishes four main powers: the medical profession, patients, the medico-industrial complex (commercial companies), and the state (government).

Figure 8.1 applies this model to the pharmaceutical industry. This allows us to identify the different relationships the industry is involved in, and explore its power in each case. For instance, the medical profession is potentially an important countervailing power and could be a major independent force. In general, however, the profession is largely supportive of the pharmaceutical industry, depending heavily on pharmacological treatments for its own power and status, as well as being subject to numerous blandishments from the industry. Similarly, governments have the potential to act as a countervailing power, regulating the industry through a range of mechanisms (see below). They can decide which drugs must be prescribed, which can be sold over the counter (OTC), and whether direct-to-consumer advertising is permitted. They can attempt to control drug prices, and determine whether products can be released onto the market. At the same time, as with the medical profession, they may be keen to support the industry because of its economic contribution, or to secure favourable access to products. Finally, patients can be a countervailing force, but their power tends to be limited unless operating collectively through users' groups.

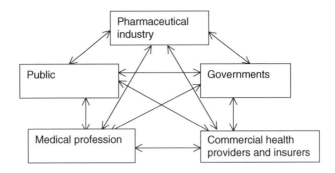

Mann's (1993) discussion of four sources of power is also useful for understanding the pharmaceutical industry. He distinguishes economic, political, ideological and military power – but only the first three apply to the pharmaceutical industry. The industry's economic power is extensive because of the scale of the industry, the high degree of consolidation, and its economic importance to the countries where major companies are located. This was apparent when the French government made its preference clear for Sanofi-Synthelabo's bid for its sister French company, Aventis, over the possible bid from the Swiss, Novartis. The industry's economic power therefore can give it attendant political power.

In addition the industry has ideological power. This operates most obviously through the marketing carried out by leading companies. This marketing activity is well-documented. In the US direct-to-consumer advertising is permitted, and there is extensive and highly effective advertising through the mass media. Studies show that the most advertised brands are the most widely prescribed. Where such advertising is banned, product marketing is still wide-ranging. Companies make considerable use of press releases about products and the illnesses they treat, often emphasizing how these illnesses often go undetected, which the mass media then pick up. Consequently, the public often learn about new products through newspapers, magazines and television. Moreover, direct marketing to doctors and other health professionals is extensive. This includes advertisements in medical publications, sponsorship of meetings and research, provision of branded items, and personal contact by sales representatives. Leading companies spend around 12% of revenue on marketing. Since regulatory controls are typically weaker in low-income countries, the potential ideological power of companies through publicity and marketing is considerable despite more limited purchasing power.

Activity 8.2

Obtain a copy of a medical journal that accepts drug advertisements. Look at the drug products advertised in it and the language used to describe them. What proportion is for leading products? Who are the manufacturers? How do the advertisements encourage the use of the different products?

Regulating the pharmaceutical industry

Regulating trade

The WTO is by far the most important organization regulating international trade, including trade in pharmaceuticals. As described in Chapter 7, it operates through periodically held trade negotiations and agreed multilateral agreements. One new area of its work, particularly relevant to the industry, is intellectual property rights. The Agreement on Trade-Related Aspects of Intellectual Property Rights (TRIPS) adopted in 1995 covers such matters as copyright, trademarks, geographical locations and patents. It is designed to protect IPR across the world, although least developed countries have until 2016 to put it fully into effect.

The agreement recognizes that patent protection can sometimes be overridden on public health grounds, for instance when there are major epidemics. In these circumstances a government may introduce 'compulsory licensing' permitting a local company to produce a patented product without the agreement of the patent owner. However, a country may do so only if they have first sought a voluntary licence from the patent holder, and must restrict use of the drug to the domestic market. The subsequent Doha Declaration, agreed in 2001, allows a country to issue a compulsory licence to import a drug from another country if there is no domestic pharmaceutical industry, although some remuneration must be paid to the exporter.

Regulating products and prices

Safety concerns about drug adulteration, and the addictive properties of some medicines, have led to the regulation of products that can be marketed, and whether they require medical prescription. Drug approval agencies only fully developed in western countries in the early 1960s, partly following the tragic consequences arising from the use of thalidomide, which heightened concerns about drug safety and effectiveness. An agency's task is to assess the benefits and risks of a drug for the treatment of a particular condition. Countries vary in the rigour of their approval agencies, and the extent to which they rely on prior judgements made by other agencies. Agencies review both patented and generic drugs before they can be released onto the market. They typically depend on the test results provided (and usually funded) by pharmaceutical companies, rather than their own research. As we would expect, the requirements for approving generic drugs are usually more limited than for drugs involving new active substances.

Drug approval agencies mediate between the conflicting interests of pharmaceutical companies, which seek to make a profit and get products onto the market as quickly as possible, and the public who, while having an interest in securing speedy access to a new treatment, also have a strong interest in effectiveness and safety. Agencies have to deal with these conflicting interests on behalf of governments, which may also be torn between their desire to support the industry and to protect patients.

Agencies differ in their organizational structures, testing requirements and assessment procedures. Among national agencies, the most important globally is the

American FDA given the importance of accessing the huge US market. The European Agency for the Evaluation of Medicinal Products (EMEA) now sets approval standards for EU countries. Its powers are presently limited, and approval is mandatory only for biotechnology and 'orphan' drugs (see below). Since the early 1990s, the International Conference on Harmonization of Technical Requirements for the Registration of Pharmaceuticals for Human Use (ICH) has been agreeing international guidelines on a range of matters concerning testing and clinical trials. It currently has representatives from the pharmaceutical associations and regulatory agencies from the EU, US and Japan. The WHO is also beginning to play a part in commenting on the safety and effectiveness of drugs through the construction of essential drug lists largely for use in low-income countries. For instance, in 2004 it withdrew its approval of three generic drugs for HIV/AIDS.

Governments and health care organizations may also seek to regulate prices. In so doing, they may be anxious not to alienate the industry, especially if there are R&D or manufacturing facilities located within the country that contribute to it's employment, wealth or tax revenue. The precise mechanisms used to determine fair prices vary, and can sometimes be seen to favour the industry.

How effective is product regulation?

In considering the adequacy of regulatory arrangements for drug approval, two questions need to be addressed: are the regulatory agencies independent of the pharmaceutical industry; and is safety and effectiveness adequately assessed before a drug is released onto the market? First, there can be a problem of *regulatory capture* whereby agencies take on the values and interests of the group whose activities it regulates. A number of factors facilitate capture. One is the difficulty of finding the necessary expertise entirely independent of the industry to make assessments. Another is the companies' power in the face of a government's desire to support the industry. Moreover, some governments are politically sympathetic to large-scale companies on ideological grounds.

Second, there are various reasons why the safety and effectiveness of drugs may not be adequately assessed before they are released onto the market. This is recognized by the regulatory agencies themselves, which accept that further evaluation will be needed once the drug is licensed for the market. However, once approval is granted there is less systematic testing of drugs using properly controlled trials. The key limitations of testing are described in Table 8.4. The consequence is that, in many cases, problems with particular medicines only emerge after they have been on the market for some time. They may be withdrawn or the advice on use changed significantly. For instance, the statin, Baycol® was voluntarily withdrawn in 2001, four years after it was first licensed in the US, after it led to 31 deaths in the US alone. The pain-reducing Vioxx®, used in the treatment of arthritis and with sales of US$2.5 billion, was withdrawn in 2004 after clinical trials identified an increased risk of heart attacks among users. Full evaluation of a drug can take many years, with many people suffering side effects and adverse drug reactions during this time.

Table 8.4 The limitations of drug testing

Limitation	Problem
1. Lack of independent testing	Most testing is funded by the industry; when research is independent results are usually less favourable to the tested drug
2. Lack of transparency over test results	Unfavourable results may not be revealed by companies under the guise of commercial confidentiality
3. Companies decide how to handle trial withdrawals	Attrition affects trial results and can be used to make a drug look more effective
4. Limited number of human subjects tested	Tests usually involve a few thousand people and uncommon side effects may not show up
5. Narrow range of human subjects	Most testing is on men and excludes women, children and the elderly, yet a drug may be used for these groups even though they have different metabolisms
6. Narrow range of cases, with clearly defined illness	Boundaries of a drug's value are not tested though the cost-benefit equation changes for more marginal cases
7. Companies select comparators and dosages to test	Can make a drug look more effective by using higher dosage of the tested drug or a low dosage of comparator
8. Companies select measures of effectiveness	Small differences that are not clinically significant can be presented as showing greater effectiveness
9. Testing mainly short-term, usually no more than 6 months	Problems with long-term use will not show up
10. Limited systematic testing of interaction effects	Drugs are often taken alongside one another, especially among older people
11. Limited post-approval testing	Need systematic research under conditions of normal clinical practice
12. Poor post-approval systems for reporting side effects and ADRs	Adverse drug reactions and side effects tend to be massively under-reported

A further issue is the use of subjects from low-income countries to test medicines to be used in high-income countries, a practice which raises major ethical issues. A classic example was the testing of the first contraceptive pill on Puerto Rican women. The practice exposes the trial subjects to the risks associated with a new product, which will often, because of its cost, have its major markets in more affluent countries and indeed may no longer be available to these individuals once the trial is completed. Finally, in countries where drug approval is less stringent, drugs withdrawn from use in high-income countries may continue to be widely marketed elsewhere. Overall, the regulatory framework for the pharmaceutical industry remains variable at the national level, and nascent at the international level. If the industry becomes more globalized (see below), this framework will need to be strengthened to appropriately balance the interests of drug companies and users.

To what extent is the pharmaceutical industry globalizing?

In considering the extent to which the pharmaceutical industry is globalizing, it is helpful to distinguish trade, manufacturing and product innovation activities in the context of the three types of economic globalization described in Chapter 6. In terms of trade, the industry can be described as 'internationalized' given the large number of companies that sell products across the world. However, as Table 8.2 indicates, the distribution of world sales revenue is imbalanced. The pharmaceuticals trade is dominated by the leading companies selling to high-income countries. Trade in generic drugs is also dominated by western companies, although there is growing trade among non-western countries and the largest non-western companies are beginning to get a foothold in western markets. The *liberalization* of trade is somewhat uneven. Various developments have opened up trade, including moves to harmonize drug approval standards (see below) and the accession of more countries to the WTO. However, whether the enforcement of IPRs facilitates or hinders trade remains subject to debate. Some argue that it constitutes a form of market imperfection on the supply side. Others believe it forms an important pillar of a global drug market.

Second, there is evidence of the internationalization of manufacturing. Although the headquarters of the ten leading companies are concentrated in a few countries, they manufacture their products in a range of countries. For example, AstraZeneca has 34 manufacturing sites in 20 countries, with principal manufacturing facilities in the UK, Sweden, US, Australia, Brazil, China, France, Germany, Italy, Japan and Puerto Rico.

Third, product innovation remains concentrated in western countries, with leading companies having perhaps one research facility elsewhere. For instance, AstraZeneca's R&D is carried out in Sweden, the UK, the US, Canada and India, the only non-western location. Pfizer's R&D is largely located in the US, but it also has important research facilities in the UK, France and Japan, the only non-western location. However, as noted above, large companies in countries like India and Brazil are increasingly investing in R&D.

Overall, it is more accurate to say that there has so far been a process of westernization rather than globalization (Table 8.5). But the situation is changing towards internationalization, as companies in China, Japan and India become more important to global markets. The industry does not yet transcend boundaries – globalization in its strictest sense – although the growing sale of drugs via the Internet may qualify as a form of transcendence.

Table 8.5 The pharmaceutical industry and globalization

Type of globalization	Extent
Internationalization – leading companies trade across the world	Pharmaceutical trade is extensive, but is largely asymmetrical flowing from the west.
Liberalization – reduction of trade barriers	Moves to harmonize drug approval standards and accession to WTO reduces trade barriers but patenting creates market imperfections.
Globalization – transcendence of boundaries	While there are signs that production is delinked from geography, on the whole consumption and product innovation are not.

The consequences of a globalizing pharmaceutical industry

There are three main issues raised by an increasingly globalized pharmaceutical industry: the role of drugs in influencing health status; the need to correct commercial biases in the supply of drugs; and the inappropriate use of medicines.

Health status

In his classic study of the factors underpinning the long-term decline in mortality from infectious diseases in Britain from 1750 to 1950, McKeown (1976) argued that new vaccines made relatively little contribution. The data for respiratory tuberculosis are given in Figure 8.2. Rather, the first stage of the demographic transition from high mortality and fertility to low mortality and fertility, predated the introduction of relevant vaccines. Instead improving living standards were crucial. Subsequent writers have suggested that other factors, such as improvements in sanitation, were more important than general living standards. Yet they do not contradict McKeown's central point that medical interventions were less important to the long-term declines in mortality associated with the demographic transition than the broader social determinants of health.

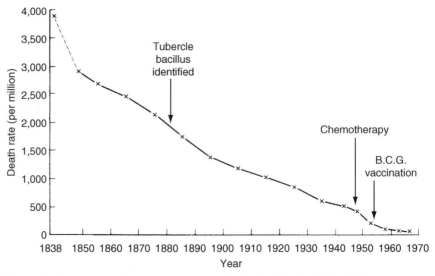

Figure 8.2 Respiratory tuberculosis death rates, England and Wales, 1838–1970
Source: McKeown (1976).

The health problems that now face high-income countries following the demographic transition are very different. Life expectancy is generally high and still increasing, and the majority of deaths result from bodily degeneration – cancers, heart disease and respiratory problems. Nonetheless the significance of social factors to health status still applies. For instance, the high levels of obesity, which now threaten health in many affluent countries, are largely the result of changes in patterns of nutrition and physical activity. It can best be tackled, therefore, by tackling these social factors (e.g. food consumption, the nature of work, modes of travel) rather than by medicines.

In low-income countries that have not yet undergone the demographic transition, infectious diseases cause a higher burden of ill-health. McKeown's analysis also supports the argument that improved living standards and social conditions, through economic development and poverty reduction, are the key to improving health. Where medical interventions are involved, preventive measures such as vaccination are equally if not more important to improving health than treatment regimes.

Notwithstanding the evidence of the importance of social factors to health status, some argue that there has been an increasing *medicalization* of problems with social origins, transforming them into health problems, a trend to which the pharmaceutical industry has contributed. This medicalization is associated with the development of new treatments and new categories of disease. This can be seen with new psychotropic medications, which have been linked with the introduction of new disease categories. As a result, aspects of behaviour that might once have been regarded as needing to be managed through care, education or social reform, tend now to be seen as indicative of mental disorder and treated with drugs. There are also concerns that the focus, in high-income countries, on treatment rather than prevention will be extended to low-income countries through globalization of drug use practices.

Attention to the broad determinants of health does not mean, of course, that drug technologies and other medical interventions do not affect health status. One study contended that about half of the increase in life expectancy in Britain since 1950 could be accounted for by medical care (Bunker, 2001), but others have argued that this is an overestimate arising from incorrect assumptions in the analysis. However, not all benefits from drugs can be captured by changes in mortality. The reduction of pain and suffering is a major motivation for the use of medicines, as the continuing popularity of aspirin and paracetamol attests. Medicines can also shorten the duration of an illness, important for the quality of life of an individual as well as to society as a whole.

Commercial biases

As commercial bodies, pharmaceutical companies concentrate on producing drugs that are potentially profitable. However, this leads to biases in product portfolios. First, drugs for chronic complaints are more attractive commercially than those for acute, shorter-term illnesses, even if life threatening. The size of the former market is potentially greater and profits higher, so drugs for chronic complaints dominate product development (see Table 8.3). Severe illnesses, such as cancers, are not entirely neglected, but drugs to treat them usually do not offer the same revenue potential. Second, rare illnesses tend to get less attention, even if very serious, given the potentially small market for treatments. The extent of this problem of so-called 'neglected diseases' has led some countries to provide specific funding to the industry to develop 'orphan' drugs for rare conditions. In the US, for example, measures were introduced in 1983 to make funding available to pharmaceutical companies for research on orphan drugs. It also introduced a procedure for getting a disease or condition formally approved as rare.

For low-income countries, the problem of commercial bias is even greater. Poorer countries have far fewer resources to spend on health care, including pharmaceuticals. Consequently, pharmaceutical companies have shown less interest in developing treatments for the health needs they face. For example, there remains a lack of effective anti-malarials, despite the disease killing around 2 million people each year in the developing world. The cost of drugs is also a major hurdle for accessing appropriate medications in developing countries. Although many of the drugs currently available are not patented, they remain beyond the resources of many low-income countries. This entails not only paying for drugs, but also the necessary infrastructure to ensure the safe and effective use of pharmaceuticals. Moreover, low-income countries are disadvantaged by the extension of IPRs. On the one hand, the cost of new, patented treatments when they emerge is prohibitive, and countries are largely prevented from producing cheaper copies. On the other hand, indigenous natural substances used in a range of medicines, from which low-income countries could benefit, are increasingly being patented by pharmaceutical companies.

HIV/AIDS is interesting in this context since it has received more attention from leading pharmaceutical companies than other diseases common in low-income countries. This is undoubtedly because the disease also affects affluent countries. Many leading companies have drugs for HIV/AIDS, but existing treatments are oriented to strains prevalent in industrialized countries. Companies protect these drugs under patents, and have been slow to make them more readily available at reduced prices or to waive patent protection. Relatively little private investment has been made to develop a vaccine for HIV/AIDS.

From an ethical perspective, it is clearly unacceptable to leave the health needs of the developing world to the profit-seeking motives of the commercial market. Moreover, neglect of these health needs is likely to prove short sighted in an increasingly globalized world where the risk of the rapid spread of infections is high. The combined use of incentives and regulation by governments and international organizations is clearly needed to address these commercial biases.

The inappropriate use of medicines

A third consequence of a globalizing pharmaceutical industry is the emergence of forces that encourage the inappropriate use of medicines. Amid increasing pressures to market drugs worldwide, a drug may be unnecessarily prescribed where, for example, an individual's condition is not sufficiently severe. Or a drug may be prescribed on the grounds that it might help, even when there is evidence that the condition is not responsive to the drug. The misuse of antibiotics for viral infections are examples having potentially global consequences in the form of growing drug resistance. Or a drug may be prescribed in a high dosage when a lower dosage would be almost as effective and have fewer side effects. Or a drug that is initially necessary may be continued for too long, increasing the chance of side effects. The indiscriminate use of medical treatment was the focus of Cochrane's (1972) classic discussion of tonsillectomy. His point was not that tonsillectomy was never effective or useful; rather he argued that the procedure was often used too freely and unnecessarily, even though it involved risks to the patient. The same argument can apply to pharmaceuticals. The globalization of the pharmaceutical market, ahead of appropriate prescribing protocols and guidelines across all countries, gives rise to individual and collective risks.

 Activity 8.3

During the past 30 years, attention deficit hyperactivity disorder and post-traumatic stress disorder have been defined by some as mental health conditions. In what ways do you think this might be described as a process of medicalization?

 Feedback

Research on these conditions is ongoing and their causes are unknown. Some argue that the fast pace of modern life, the increased exposure of children to computer games, and the increased consumption of foods containing artificial additives, may all partially explain the apparent increased incidence of attention deficit hyperactivity. It is also postulated by some that post traumatic stress may, in part be explained by the increased targeting of civilian populations caught up in conflict situations or to greater exposure to traumatizing experiences as a result of changes in lifestyle (e.g. travel to conflict zones).

Summary

You have seen how the pharmaceutical industry has undergone significant change in recent decades, with ownership consolidated into a relatively small number of large companies with increasingly global reach. The products they develop and sell, and the regulatory bodies that control this process, have consequently experienced important changes. Efforts to improve global health requires understanding of these changes, and how the pharmaceutical industry can support or hinder this goal.

References

Bunker, JP (2001) 'The role of medical care in contributing to health improvements within societies'. *International Journal of Epidemiology*, 30: 1260–3.

Cochrane AL (1972) *Effectiveness and Efficiency: Random Reflections on Health Services*. London: Nuffield Provincial Hospitals Trust.

IMS Health (2002) 'IMS launches world review for generic pharmaceutical industry'. http://open.imshealth.com/webshop2/IMSinclude/I_article_20020926a.asp, accessed 2 October 2004.

IMS Health (2004a) 'Sweetened bid from Sanofi-Synthelabo wins Aventis'. http://open.imshealth.com/webshop2/IMSinclude/1_article_20040130a.asp, accessed 27 July 2004.

IMS Health (2004b) 'IMS highlights biotech as strong growth driver'. http://open.imshealth.com/webshop2/IMSinclude/I_article_20040623.asp, accessed 3 August 2004.

IMS Health (2004c) 'Generics flourish as innovation stalls'. www.ims-global.com/insight/news_story_0406/news_story_040614a.htm, accessed 27 July 2004.

IMS Health (2004d) 'Top companies, July 2004' http://open.imshealth.com/dept.asp/dept%5Fid=2.

IMS Health (2004e) '2003 global pharma sale by region' www.ims-global.com/insight/news_story_040316.htm.

IMS Health (2004e) 'Lipitor leads the way in 2003' www.ims-global.com/insight/news_story/0403/news_story_040316.htm.

Kaiser Family Foundation (2004) 'Trends and indicators in the changing health care marketplace, 2004 update'. http://www.kff.org/insurance/7031/t12004–1–21.cfm, accessed 4 September 2004.

Light D (1995) 'Countervailing powers: a framework for professions in transition'. In *Health Professions and the State in Europe*. (Johnson T, Larkin G and Saks M, eds). London: Routledge.

McKeown T (1976) *The Modern Rise of Population*. London: Edward Arnold.

Mann, M (1993) *The Sources of Social Power, Vol II, The Rise of Classes and Nation States, 1760–1914*. Cambridge: Cambridge University Press.

NIHCM (2002) *Changing Patterns of Pharmaceutical Innovation*. Washington: National Institute for Health Care Management Foundation.

Tarabusi C and Vickery G (1998) 'Globalization in the pharmaceutical industry, Parts I and II'. *International Journal of Health Services*, 28: 67–105, 282–303.

9 The global economy and the tobacco pandemic

Overview

In this chapter you will learn about the rapidly changing structure of the tobacco industry, which provides a clear example of the broader shift from an international to a global economy as described in Chapter 6. Such an analysis of the tobacco industry offers valuable insights into the relationship between global change and health. Given the sheer scale of tobacco's impact on health, evidence of how key aspects of political and economic change have facilitated tobacco companies' global expansion assumes particular significance. Traditional forms of health governance have been demonstrated to be incapable of effectively responding to the threat posed by the tobacco industry, a recognition that has given rise to a unique initiative. The Framework Convention on Tobacco Control, WHO's first attempt to negotiate an international public health treaty, is presented here as an attempt to regulate the activities of transnational tobacco companies.

Learning objectives

After working through this chapter, you should be able to:

- outline recent developments in the tobacco pandemic and its implications for health equity
- understand the impact of trade liberalization on tobacco consumption
- assess the distinctive threats to global health posed by transnational tobacco companies
- explain the emergence of WHO's Framework Convention on Tobacco Control
- consider how different aspects of global change pose opportunities and threats for effective responses to the tobacco pandemic.

Key terms

Smoking prevalence The percentage of a given population that currently smoke tobacco.

Trade liberalization The process by which national economies become more open to cross-border flows of goods, services and capital.

Tobacco and global health

Consumption of cigarettes and other tobacco products and exposure to tobacco smoke collectively constitute the world's leading preventable cause of deaths in adults, being responsible for around 5 million deaths per year (WHO, 2003) or approximately one in 10 of all adult deaths. The global scale of tobacco's health impacts merits the use of the term pandemic, and this pandemic is undergoing rapid acceleration. Mortality levels attributable to tobacco have increased by around 45% since 1990, and are expected to double to around 10 million p.a. (or one in six adult deaths) by 2030 unless widespread and effective interventions are rapidly implemented.

The global distribution of tobacco consumption is also undergoing rapid change, and its diverse social, economic and health impacts are becoming increasingly inequitable. A broad decline in smoking prevalence across most high-income countries in recent decades has coincided with substantial increases among low- and middle-income countries. Given the lengthy delay between the onset of smoking and tobacco's health impacts, this global shift is being slowly but inexorably followed by a redistribution of tobacco-related disease and death.

- An estimated 82% of the world's smokers live in low and middle income countries;
- About half of all tobacco-related deaths now occur in those countries;
- By 2030 low- and middle-income countries will account for around seven in 10 of all tobacco-related deaths;
- In China, annual tobacco deaths are expected to reach 1 million before 2010 and 2 million by 2025;
- In India, around 80 million India males under the age of 35 will eventually be killed by tobacco (Thun and da Costa e Silva, 2003).

Within this overall shift in the tobacco pandemic there predictably exists enormous diversity among developing countries, and the pandemic remains strongly differentiated by, *inter alia*, region and gender. Driven by the huge Chinese market, consumption is estimated to be highest in the Western Pacific. While consumption remains lowest in Africa, particularly sub-Saharan Africa, the limited data currently available suggest that smoking in Africa is rising significantly, especially among the young.

While smoking prevalence among men and women have substantially converged across much of Europe and North America, huge gender disparities persist in patterns of tobacco use among developing countries. World Bank estimates smoking prevalence in high income countries at 38% for men and 21% for women, with higher rates for men and lower rates for women in low- and middle-income countries at 49% and 9% respectively. China provides a powerful illustration of this gender gap, with adult male smoking prevalence of 53.4% contrasting with only 4% among women. The scale of this divide may, however, be exaggerated as traditional cultural norms against women smoking encourage under-reporting and since the primary emphasis on cigarette smoking often ignores traditional widely practised non-commercial forms of tobacco use. In India, for example, female cigarette use in urban centres is between 2% and 5%, while up to 67% of women in rural areas use smokeless tobacco (Samet and Yoon, 2001).

Though national patterns of tobacco consumption and its health impacts continue to differ widely, they can be considered to be following broadly comparable trajectories. A four stage model developed for WHO (Lopez et al., 1994) offers a conceptual framework within which the evolution of national epidemics can be related to the broader pandemic (Figure 9.1). The key characteristics of each stage can be summarized as:

- *Stage 1* – low prevalence of cigarette smoking at under 20%, largely confined to males, while rates of lung cancer or other chronic diseases caused by smoking have not yet demonstrably increased;
- *Stage 2* – smoking prevalence among men exceeds 50%, evidence of increases among women, younger initiation, and an increasing burden of tobacco-related disease among men;
- *Stage 3* – convergence of male and female smoking prevalence given a clear reduction among men and a more gradual decline among women, but the long time lag in tobacco's health impacts result in smoking attributable mortality reaching 10% to 30% of all deaths;
- *Stage 4* – marked reductions in both male and female smoking prevalence, and smoking attributable deaths peak at 30% to 35% among men before declining, while such deaths rise to 20% to 25% of all deaths among women.

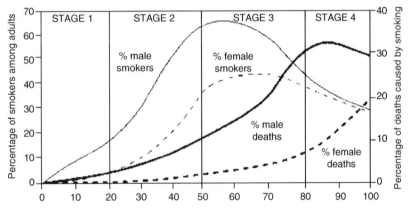

Figure 9.1 Four stages of the tobacco epidemic

Source: Thun and da Costa e Silva, 2003.

✎ **Activity 9.1**

On the basis of the WHO model described above and depicted in Figure 9.1, try to allocate a country or region to each of the four stages of the tobacco epidemic.

Feedback

> Sub-Saharan Africa is the region that most clearly exhibits the attributes of Stage 1;
> China, Japan, Southeast Asia, Latin America and North Africa broadly fit with Stage 2;
> Eastern Europe and Southern Europe can be characterized as being in Stage 3; Western
> Europe, US, Canada and Australia can be identified among those countries in Stage 4.

While tobacco clearly constitutes a global health problem, this exercise demonstrates the diversity that continues to characterize national experiences of the pandemic. Such diversity has important implications for the future development of the tobacco industry as the evolution of national epidemics is shaped by tobacco companies and impacts on their profitability. You should consider such implications as you progress through the remainder of this chapter.

Globalization and transnational tobacco companies

There is nothing novel about a link between globalization and tobacco consumption. Indeed this link can be traced back to 1492, before which tobacco use was restricted to the indigenous peoples of the Americas. Within 150 years of Columbus describing 'great multitudes of people, men and women with firebrands in their hands and herbs to smoke after their custom', tobacco was being used around the world, albeit to an often limited extent. While the geographical scope of tobacco use has long been extensive, the contemporary scale of its mass use and related health impacts are much more recent. The current pandemic represents the outcome of the huge changes arising from the development of automated cigarette rolling machines in the late nineteenth century. The cigarette was to become established as arguably the most successful commercial product of the twentieth century.

Importantly for global health, however, it appears that the commercial potential of the cigarette has not yet been fully realized. Key features of the global political economy have already effected a transformation in the structure and prospects of the tobacco industry, creating enormous commercial opportunities while exacerbating impacts on global health.

The increasingly inequitable burden of tobacco consumption owes much to the recent global expansion of a handful of transnational tobacco companies (TTCs) that are now clearly established as the primary vectors of the tobacco pandemic:

- Four companies now control around three-quarters of the global cigarette market;
- Domestic sales by China's national tobacco monopoly account for around a third of global cigarette sales;
- Philip Morris, part of the Altria group and owner of the Marlboro brand, is considered international market leader with around 16.5% of global market share;
- British American Tobacco (BAT), historically the most international and diverse tobacco company, consolidated its second position by merging with Rothmans and accounts for 15% of the world cigarette market;

- Japan Tobacco International (JTI), half owned by Japan's government, obtained third place with 8% global share after purchasing the international business of RJ Reynolds, including the Camel and Winston brands;
- The combined net revenue of these three TTCs nears $100 billion p.a., surpassing the gross national income of all but the world's 35 richest countries (WHO, 2004; *Tobacco Journal International, 2002*).

It is important to emphasize the scale of the recent changes in the profile of the global tobacco industry. Philip Morris, for example, saw its global revenues increase by 226% to US$27.4 billion from 1989–99, during which time the comparative profitability of its domestic and international tobacco operations was transformed. As Figure 9.2 demonstrates, whereas in the late 1980s PM's tobacco business in the US was about four times as profitable as its international operations, this ratio was almost reversed by 1998 (WHO, 2004).

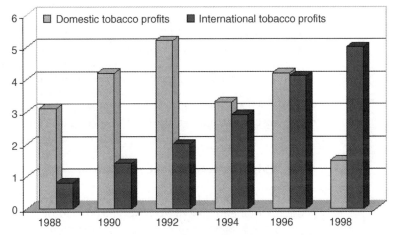

Figure 9.2 Philip Morris – profits from tobacco 1988–1998
Source: WHO, 2004.

From a global health perspective, it is particularly important to note that trade liberalization has been demonstrated to have inequitable impacts, exacerbating the global shift in the tobacco pandemic. Trade liberalization has led to:

- an overall increase in tobacco consumption;
- a large and significant impact on smoking in low income countries;
- a significant, if smaller, impact on middle income countries;
- no substantive impact on tobacco consumption in higher income countries (Taylor et al., 2000).

Pressure on TTCs' traditional bases of profitability in North America and Western Europe has increased in recent decades from the combined threats of regulation, declining consumption and litigation. Developments in the global political economy have, however, created substantial new opportunities in what TTCs refer to as emerging markets. Among key drivers of recent global expansion can be identified:

- post-cold war regime change in the former Soviet Union and Eastern Europe;
- inclusion of tobacco under the Uruguay round of GATT negotiations;
- decline and privatization of previously state-owned tobacco monopolies, encouraged by the IMF;
- increased integration of large Asian markets with the global economy.

TTCs quickly recognized the opportunities inherent in such changes. BAT's then chairman Sir Patrick Sheehy noted in 1993 that 'the tobacco markets open to our products have actually tripled in size in recent years, under the twin impact of market liberalisations across the northern hemisphere and the crumbling of monolithic communism east of the river Elbe' (Sheehy, 1993). Such opportunities triggered a major shift in corporate strategy across the TTCs from the extensive diversification of the 1980s to reinvestment in tobacco. This shift is reflected in an estimated 141 acquisitions by and mergers among major tobacco companies between 1990 and 2001 (Physicians for a Smoke-Free Canada, 2001).

Such changes are of direct relevance to health since post-privatization restructuring and the entry of TTCs into new markets are usually associated with increased tobacco consumption (WHO, 2004). This is powerfully demonstrated by the impacts of TTCs on consumption in Japan, South Korea, Taiwan and Thailand, where access to previously closed markets was gained following the threat of trade sanctions by the US (and, in the Thai case, adjudication by GATT). Average per capita cigarette consumption across these countries increased by an estimated 10% by 1991, an increase that may be explained by the lower prices and more aggressive marketing behaviour that is the likely result of increased competition.

Case study: Thailand, tobacco and trade

Since 1966 Thailand's tobacco market had been essentially closed to foreign competition; the importation of cigarettes and other tobacco products were prohibited, enabling the dominance of domestic cigarettes produced by the Thailand Tobacco Monopoly (TTM). Encouraged by the United States Cigarette Exports Association that had been formed by cigarette manufacturers Philip Morris, RJ Reynolds and Brown & Williamson, the US Trade Representative threatened retaliatory sanctions against Thailand if this prohibition was not lifted. In 1989, the United States complained that the import restrictions were inconsistent with GATT Article XI and considered that they could not be justified by either:

(i) some of the exceptions to the elimination of quantitative restrictions allowed under Art. XI, or
(ii) the 'General Exceptions' allowed by Article XX(b) pertaining to measures necessary for the protection of human life or health.

Thailand responded by arguing that the import restrictions were justified under Article XX(b) since measures adopted by the government could only be effective if cigarette imports were prohibited, while certain chemicals and additives contained in US cigarettes could be more harmful to human health than TTM products.

Submissions made to the GATT arbitration panel by WHO confirmed differences between cigarettes manufactured in developed and developing countries, with US cigarettes containing more additives and flavouring that made them easier to smoke, particularly by women and adolescents. WHO could not, however, present scientific evidence demonstrating that such cigarettes were intrinsically more harmful.

The GATT panel determined that Thailand's import restrictions were indeed inconsistent with Article XI and were not justified under either of the exceptions outlined above. Import restrictions were concluded to be unnecessary since other measures could be used to protect public health without favouring domestic production. Such alternative measures included bans on advertising. The panel therefore rejected a request from the United States that Thailand's recent ban on tobacco advertising should be lifted. With an advertising ban at the centre of extensive health regulation of tobacco, Thailand has subsequently been comparatively successful in restricting tobacco consumption.

Activity 9.2

Given the precedent of the Thailand GATT case, and based on what you learned about WTO agreements in Chapter 7, briefly identify ways in which the following health measures might conflict with the TBT, GATS and TRIPS agreements:

1 Prohibiting 'misleading descriptors' on tobacco products (i.e. use of terms like 'light' and 'mild' which have been perceived as suggesting reduced risk.
2 Requiring full public disclosure of ingredients, additives and flavourings for each cigarette brand.
3 Enlarged dramatic warnings on packaging that make health impacts more prominent while reducing the visual appeal of the brand.
4 Fully comprehensive advertising bans that cover brand sharing (developing alternative products bearing the name of tobacco advertising), sponsorships and point of sale promotions (in-store displays) in addition to traditional forms of advertising (e.g. cinema, radio, television or newspaper advertisements.

Feedback

1 This could be viewed as a violation of company trademarks. Japan has repeatedly threatened to challenge a European Union directive prohibiting such terminology (Mild Seven is a key international brand for JTI). Such a measure could conceivably be viewed as infringing either the TBT or TRIPS agreements.

2 Compulsory ingredient disclosure could impinge on the protections to product information offered by TRIPS. Yet such measures are increasingly viewed as important both in enabling consumers to make informed decisions and in allowing the future development of more effective means of regulating the composition of such harmful products.

3 Stringent requirements on packaging and labelling could be interpreted as incompatible with the protections offered by the TBT agreements.

4 While the GATT arbitration panel upheld Thai legislation it has been argued that a different verdict might now be reached under GATS, particularly in a case where such fully comprehensive prohibitions were envisaged.

Such interpretations should be viewed with caution in the absence of clear precedents. It does, however, seem reasonable to expect that at least some of these tensions are likely to be explored in the near future. The Thai case is particularly instructive since it serves to demonstrate how trade agreements can mitigate against measures that might reasonably be viewed as protecting health, while also highlighting the substantial scope remaining for effective regulation.

Globalization and tobacco: the cognitive dimension

The effects of global change are much more diverse than can be addressed by a narrowly economic conception of globalization. While trade liberalization has been particularly important to the recent trajectory of the tobacco industry, the global expansion of TTCs also highlights their appreciation of the cognitive dimension of globalization. TTCs are powerful agents of social change, actively working to shape our perceptions and conduct as, *inter alia*, consumers (actual or potential), investors, voters or regulators.

This is an aspect of globalization in which tobacco companies have been actively interested. In 1992, BAT's head of marketing Jimmi Rembiszewski gave a key-note conference speech entitled 'Think Global – Act Global – Adapt Local'. In it he traced the globalization of young people's habits and practices or lifestyle back to the late 1960s, suggesting that such globalization 'crosses not only continents but also generations'. Importantly, however, Rembiszewski emphasizes that effective commercial exploitation of such trends also needs to acknowledge their limitations:

> 'This is an area where most multinationals made mistakes when extending food brands globally. While habits and practices could be altered over time . . . *dramatic change in national taste* has been slow . . . MacDonalds in Far East taste different to Europe and most of food products (which became successful) had to be adapted to the local taste . . . Also the cigarette industry had to go through this experience. So you will find today that most international brands do have consistent advertising strategies and executions, pack designs and family line. But varying taste tailored to the local acceptance.'

The cognitive dimension of globalization offers significant opportunities to the TTCs, and they have been typically assiduous in their efforts to exploit them.

Towards the global smoker

Across key Asian markets, in particular, displacing traditional forms of tobacco such as bidis, kreteks and chewing tobacco represent an enormous potential market for expansion by the TTCs. Conversion to western-style white stick cigarettes represents a key part of the ambition to create what can be termed the 'global smoker'. An industry journal has described the continuing predominance of alternative products within such markets as India and Indonesia as illustrating the contemporary limits of globalization, but notes that such limits are being aggressively targeted:

'For how long will these markets resist the attraction of global trends? In one or two generations, the sons and grandsons of today's Indians may not want to smoke bidis or chew pan masala. Cigarette manufacturers seem not to be asking if, but how fast these markets will change. Global brands are one way to accelerate this process'. (Crescenti, 1999)

The perceived 'transnationality' of the western-style white stick cigarette has itself provided a key resource for increasing market share. The rise of cigarette sales, for example, has been presented as an indicator of modernity and symbol of economic progress within low-income countries. A letter from the India Tobacco Company urged the Minister of Health to 'encourage a conversion to cigarettes, which is the internationally accepted form of tobacco use' (Chugh, 1992). Such promotion has entailed inferences of personal prestige and veiled health claims. In Indonesia, a BAT study of smokers of global brands found that one of the perceived advantages of white cigarettes was that 'it is less dangerous to health' (BAT Indonesia, no date). The attempt to associate cigarettes with western and, particularly, American images of freedom and prosperity is widespread. In the Czech Republic, for example, an advertisement for L&M cigarettes features a picture of the pack alongside the Statue of Liberty with a slogan translating as 'This is what America tastes like! New Arrival!'

Developing global brands

Premium international brands constitute the fastest growing portion of the world cigarette market with annual sales growing at about 5% during the 1990s. They are of key strategic significance to TTCs since they offer higher prices, production volumes, economies of scale and, crucially, opportunities to coherently build perceptions of a brand on a cross-national basis. For BAT:

'International brands are defined as those brands that are available in a number of markets and currently sell, or have the potential to sell, significant volumes in the future. They are generally priced at a higher or premium level, have consistent pack designs and communications to the smoker with a clear target consumer in mind . . . The fact that a "foreign" brand is sold on another market is not sufficient to justify its description as an International Brand, because the latter involves a mix of global availability, plus perception of internationality to the consumer'. (BATCo, 1994)

The template for this strategy was set by Philip Morris's success in transforming Marlboro from a stagnant American brand in the early 1960s, to a business phenomenon and one of the handful of truly global brands. Marlboro continues to dwarf its competitors, accounting for 8.4% of global cigarette consumption, a success that is inseparable from the brilliance and ubiquity of its advertising and marketing. The Marlboro Man was declared by *Advertising Age* to be the number one advertising icon of the twentieth century, and the campaign transformed the fortunes of the brand. It established a strong image that has been applied consistently across markets, with minor adaptations to accommodate local norms.

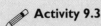

Activity 9.3

The diverse promotional activities undertaken by tobacco companies are directed at differing audiences and, in combination, pursue multiple objectives. Make a brief list of the strategic advantages that might be offered by:

1   an international sport sponsorship, such as Formula One motor racing;
2   a campaign to eliminate the use of child labour in tobacco production;

Give attention to the regulatory environment in which tobacco companies have to operate, where conventional forms of advertising are increasingly denied to them.

Feedback

1 Sports sponsorship has assumed increasing importance as advertising restrictions have been tightened. Crucially, they typically serve to maintain a television presence for cigarette brands, while sports sponsorship can also tie brands to hugely popular individuals or teams. Different sports fit a range of marketing needs, but motor sports are particularly useful because they offer tobacco companies control over the visual aspects of the sport (i.e. the colours of racing cars and drivers' uniforms can match those of the sponsoring brand). International sponsorships can also serve to promote the global expansion of a brand and to further weaken health legislation, since even bans on sponsorship can be undermined by the beaming back of television images from events in countries without such regulation. Sponsorship can also serve to exert political influence both via the creation of influential allies (e.g. sports organizations and ruling bodies) and opportunities for hospitality, allowing discussion with regulators in a relaxed environment.

2 The Elimination of Child Labour in Tobacco Growing Foundation was formed in 2001. BAT was instrumental in its formation, and all of the world's leading cigarette manufacturers and tobacco leaf companies are now members. A key strategic challenge confronting tobacco companies is the need to rebuild their reputations so as to secure their long-term viability on investment markets and reduce the political pressure for ever more extensive legislation. This need explains why corporate social responsibility has been so enthusiastically embraced by tobacco companies. The interest in eliminating child labour is strategically well chosen since it appears to demonstrate a responsible commitment to the well-being of the societies in which tobacco companies operate, and therefore is politically valuable among producer countries and might serve to reduce criticism of TTCs by international NGOs.

Negotiating the framework convention on tobacco control

A text laboriously developed following two preliminary meetings of a working group and across six sessions of an Intergovernmental Negotiating Body (INB) received the unanimous endorsement of the 56th World Health Assembly in May 2003. This concluded four years of negotiations for a Framework Convention on Tobacco Control (FCTC), WHO's first attempt to exercise its constitutional authority to develop a global public health treaty. Based on recognition of the challenges posed by globalization, the FCTC is intended to create an international public health movement capable both of addressing transnational issues and of providing a powerful resource in support of national health efforts and. Among the key features of the final text are provisions encouraging countries to:

- enact comprehensive bans on tobacco advertising, promotion and sponsorship;
- require large rotating health warnings on packaging, to cover at least 30% of principal display areas, and with provision for pictorial warnings;
- prohibit the use of misleading descriptors such as 'light' or 'mild';
- increase taxation of tobacco products;
- provide greater protection from involuntary exposure to tobacco smoke;
- develop measures to combat smuggling.

The FCTC text is lacking in binding obligations, which may be developed further by a number of issue-specific protocols, and failed to include language that would clarify its status in relationship to existing trade agreements ('health vs. trade' being the single most divisive issue during negotiations). Such caveats notwith-standing, however, the final text was both broadly welcomed by health groups and a remarkable advance on the heavily criticized preceding draft.

The significance of the FCTC, however, arguably resides primarily in the process of its development rather than in the content of the text.

Support of UN organizations and the World Bank

A key task for WHO in enabling the development of the FCTC was to secure the acquiescence, of other international agencies with an interest in tobacco issues. An initial step was the establishment in 1999 of the Ad Hoc Inter-Agency Task Force on Tobacco Control to improve coordination and cooperation. WHO was awarded leadership of the task force, signalling a shift by UN agencies towards primarily viewing tobacco issues from a health perspective. The work of the Task Force engaged the participation of 15 UN organizations as well as the World Bank, the International Monetary Fund and the WTO.

The increasing engagement of the World Bank was of critical importance in enabling the FCTC process, and particularly in building support among developing countries. A landmark here was the World Bank's publication of the 1999 report *Curbing the Epidemic*, depicting comprehensive tobacco control measures as providing a virtuous circle of cost-effectiveness and impacts on health:

> 'Policies that reduce the demand for tobacco, such as a decision to increase tobacco taxes, would not cause long term job losses in the vast majority of countries. Nor would higher tobacco taxes reduce tax revenues; rather, revenues would climb in the medium term. Such policies could, in sum, bring unprece-dented health benefits without harming economies'. (Jha and Chaloupka, 1999)

This report has been critical in undermining the widespread belief in the existence of net economic benefits from tobacco production and consumption, the perva-siveness of which has historically constituted the single greatest political obstacle to the progress of effective regulation. It is also worth noting the tobacco industry's internal recognition of the significance of Brundtland's ability to attract active support from the World Bank to the FCTC's prospects of success (BAT, no date).

Extensive participation by WHO member states

While concerned to make the FCTC process broadly inclusive, the primary focus of an international organization such as WHO was inevitably on engaging the support of its member states. Here the level of involvement throughout a protracted process was impressive, albeit characterized by predictable inequalities across national delegations in terms of their scale and breadth of expertise. Resolution 52.18 was unanimously adopted by the World Health Assembly in 1999, when a record 50 states took the floor to commit political and economic support. The first Intergovernmental Negotiating Body in October 2000 was attended by 148 countries, while the final round of negotiations in February 2003 involved delegations from 171 countries. Importantly, the demands of attendance and participation have required an expanded role for multisectoral collaboration on tobacco issues at the national level. For example, formal and informal committees have been established and regular inter-ministerial consultations have been held, often for the first time, in countries as diverse as Zimbabwe, China, Brazil, Thailand and the US.

The persistent leadership exercised by developing countries in pressing for a strong FCTC was rapidly established as a distinguishing feature of the FCTC negotiations, and this does much to explain the strength of the eventual text. This leadership role reflects political decisions made both to shape the agenda and to cope with the onerous demands of the protracted sessions of the INB in Geneva. Delegates from WHO's African region were the first to participate as a regional bloc. Anticipated divisions between tobacco producing and non-producing countries were avoided by developing common positions at preparatory meetings prior to each INB. Such positions were widely viewed as heightening the impact of African countries on the negotiations and the practice was subsequently adopted by other regions. In turn, this facilitated the development of cross-regional alliances, most significantly that between the African and South-East Asian regions.

By contrast, a minimalist FCTC incorporating aspirations rather than obligations was consistently advocated by a small number of countries where transnational tobacco companies were particularly influential. These included Japan and Germany, but the United States emerged as their most prominent proponent, particularly (thought not exclusively) following the election of the Bush administration. Democrat Congressman Henry Waxman published articles and letters highlighting the administration's efforts to undermine FCTC negotiations. These included claims that, following a meeting with representatives of Philip Morris, US negotiators pursued 10 of 11 requested deletions from proposed text (Waxman, 2002). Additionally, a leaked memo from the US Embassy in Riyadh urged Saudi Arabian assistance in backing US efforts to manage the debate around the relationship between trade and health, encouraging the attendance of delegates from economic ministries to ensure that the perspective of the health department was not unchallenged.

Corporate documents from BAT also indicate the scale of industry efforts to influence the negotiation process. An internal document from BAT described the FCTC as 'an unprecedented challenge to the tobacco industry's freedom to continue doing business', accepted that an agreement was likely and established a strategy for minimizing its potential impact. Seeking to build support among potentially sympathetic states, health and finance ministers were to be targeted as 'our priority stakeholders', while growers, unions and trade organizations were also identified as potentially useful. The document claimed 'some success at governmental level' in stimulating favourable contributions to the drafting process by Brazil, China, Germany, Argentina and Zimbabwe (BAT, no date). Additionally, tobacco companies were sporadically successful in ensuring that their representatives formed part of negotiating delegations.

The FCTC and civil society

The FCTC process also entailed efforts to include civil society, efforts that were necessarily partial and a predictable source of tension within a fundamentally essentially state-centric policy process. The terms of participation of NGOs remained strongly contested throughout the negotiation process, but there were some moves to ease or accelerate these narrow parameters. Following an open consultation held by Canada and Thailand, member states approved recommendations to accelerate the process of accreditation and allow NGOs in official relations access to open working groups. WHO's Executive Board also agreed to admit NGOs into provisional official relations with the WHO, a status that would be revised yearly throughout the FCTC process.

An innovative exercise in granting a voice to civil society organizations (CSOs) was the holding of public hearings in October 2000, the first time WHO had undertaken such an exercise. Though clearly a limited form of informal participation, and arguably primarily a sop to tobacco manufacturers and producers bemoaning their exclusion from the FCTC process, it did enable a total of 144 organizations to provided oral testimony, while 500 written submissions were received.

The involvement of CSOs in the FCTC process was greatly enhanced by the formation and development of the Framework Convention Alliance (FCA). At the two working group meetings that preceded the formal negotiations of the INB, civil society participation had been largely confined to high-income country NGOs and international health-based NGOs. By February 2003 the FCA encompassed more than 180 NGOs from over 70 countries, and had established itself as an important lobbying alliance. Coordinated via the FCA, NGOs in official relations with WHO were able to exploit their limited access to fulfil significant lobbying, educational and monitoring roles. The expertise accumulated within the FCA became a key resource, particularly in progressive alliance with the African and South-East Asian regions. Additionally, a few prominent advocates were occasionally included within the official delegations of member states.

The impact of civil society in the final negotiations was, however, significantly hampered by increasing unease among member states opposed to a powerful text. The designation of most negotiating sessions of the final INB as informal provided a simple mechanism for the exclusion of NGO participants; a reduction of access and transparency reportedly supported by delegations including the US and China.

Activity 9.4

How significant is the Framework Convention on Tobacco Control as an innovation in global health governance?

Feedback

The convention is widely regarded as a comparatively impressive document, incorporating more substantial commitments than many anticipated. Its impact on health will, however, be dependent on widespread adoption by states, effective implementation at national level, and on whether there exists the political will for the further negotiation of protocols (requiring more specific obligations). Of greater significance than the FCTC itself, however, are likely to be the multiple and diverse impacts of the process of its negotiation. As an innovation in global health governance, it represents a partial opening to non-state actors. Civil society groups played important roles but their participation was circumscribed, while the official involvement of TTCs in the process was restricted to the public hearings. Beyond its significance as a tobacco control measure, the FCTC assumes broader relevance as a response to the restricted capacity of national governance to effectively address global health risks. It can also be viewed as a unique effort to regulate the conduct of transnational corporations.

Summary

You have learned how the FCTC stands as a demonstration of a countervailing force to the tobacco industry. The cognitive dimension of globalization has, for example, been extensively exploited in countering the tobacco pandemic. The adoption of regulation in one jurisdiction has repeatedly been followed by the rapid spread of similar policies. You have seen how the widespread emergence of litigation as a tool in tobacco control similarly reflects the perceived success of such strategies within the US.

References

BAT Indonesia (no date) 'A Study on the Smokers of International Brands', Guildford Depository, Bates No.: 400458935–9056.

BATCo Marketing Intelligence Department (1994) 'International Brands 1988–1992', Guildford Depository, January, Bates No.: 500056134–6179.

British American Tobacco (no date) *British American Tobacco: Proposed WHO Tobacco Free Initiative Strategy.*

Chugh K (1992) 'Letter to Honourable Shri ML Fotedar MP, Union Minister for Health, India, Re: Tobacco Policy and the Example of Japan', Guildford Depository, 22 December, Bates No.: 304046975–6981.

Crescenti M (1999) 'The New Tobacco World'. *Tobacco Journal International*, (March), 51–3.

http://www.publici.org/download/fctc/BAT_Proposed_WHO_TFI_Strategy.pdf

Jha P and Chaloupka F (1999) *Curbing the Epidemic: Governments and the Economics of Tobacco Control*. Washington DC: World Bank.

Lopez A, Collishaw N and Piha T (1994) 'A descriptive model of the cigarette epidemic in developed countries'. *Tobacco Control*, 3: 242–7.

Physicians for a Smoke-Free Canada (2001) *An Introduction to International Trade Agreements and Their Impact on Public Measures to Reduce Tobacco Use*. April.

Rembiszewski J (1992) 'Think Global – Act Global – Adapt Local' Speech, BSB Dorland Annual conference, Guildford Depository, Bates No: 500062031–2040.

Samet J and Yoon S, eds (2001) *Women and the Tobacco Epidemic: Challenges for the 21st Century*. Geneva: World Health Organization.

Sheehy P (1993) Speech to the Farmers President's Council Meeting, British American Tobacco, Guildford Depository, 8 June, Bates No.: 601023526–3540.

Taylor A, Chaloupka F, Guindon E and Corbett M (2000) 'The impact of trade liberalization on tobacco consumption'. In *Tobacco Control in Developing Countries* (Jha P and Chaloupka F, eds). Oxford: Oxford University Press: 343–64.

Thun M and da Costa e Silva VL (2003) 'Introduction and Overview of Global Tobacco Surveillance'. In *Tobacco Control Country Profiles*. Second Edition. (Shafey O, Dolwick S and Guindon GE, eds). Atlanta, GA: American Cancer Society.

World Health Organization (2003) *The World Health Report 2003; Shaping the Future*. Geneva: WHO.

World Health Organization (2004) *Building Blocks for Tobacco Control: A Handbook*. Geneva: WHO.

Global environmental changes, climate change and human health

Overview

In this chapter you will explore the health impacts of global environmental changes (GEC). This is a complex and rather technical subject. You will begin by examining GEC, how it relates to globalization (a mix of economic, social, cultural, technological, physical and other changes), and the sorts of health impacts it might have, both now and in future. This topic's unusual spatial and temporal framework, extending globally and over the coming century, raises questions about how the GEC-health relationship relates to sustainability. In the second part of the chapter you will consider the types of public health research that can be conducted to identify current and future health risks from GEC. You will examine specific examples of such research in relation to global climate change.

Learning objectives

After working through this chapter, you will be able to:

- **distinguish global environmental changes (GEC) in general from more traditional environmental hazards**
- **understand the basic process, causes and manifestations of climate change**
- **understand how GEC relate to sustainability**
- **recognize the ways in which climate change, directly and indirectly, affects human health**
- **understand some of the difficulties in estimating the health impacts of climate change.**

Key terms

Adaptation An action (or spontaneous change) that lessens the adverse impacts of GEC.

Biodiversity The natural range of species (or intra-species genetic strains) within an ecosystem which provides a source of resilience, stability and productivity.

Carrying capacity The size of population that can be indefinitely supported by the natural resource base of the specified geographic area.

Climate change Long-term change (over decades, centuries or millennia) in average meteorological conditions (such as temperature and rainfall).

Climate variability Shifts in climatic patterns that are relatively short-term (over years or decades) but that go beyond individual weather events.

Global environmental change Large-scale human-induced changes in the Earth's natural environment in recent decades as a reflection of unprecedented impacts on the biosphere.

Scenario A description of a set of conditions, either now or, plausibly, in the future.

Weather Day-to-day climatic conditions versus longer-term conditions that define a prevailing *climate*.

Understanding global environmental change

Humans (like other species) depend upon the biosphere's complex geophysical and ecological systems to sustain their health and survival. This natural environment not only provides air, food and water, it provides a range of life-supporting environmental 'goods' (e.g. clothing materials, shelter and energy) and 'services' (e.g. constancy of local climate, pollination of food plants, and uptake of carbon dioxide and production of oxygen via plant photosynthesis).

Over many millennia, human societies have found ways to increase the 'carrying capacity' of their local environment by modifying it, exploiting local resources, and supplementing local food supplies and other materials via trade. This (in the shorter term) has been a triumph of human culture. Human societies have moved from a hunter-gatherer existence, to agrarianism (coupled increasingly with urban living), then to industrialization, and today to a post-industrial 'information age'. Each such change has required a trade-off between the resultant increase in human population density (via gains in environmental carrying capacity), and longer-term weakening of the local environment's life-supporting capacity (McMichael, 2001).

The historical record suggests that failure to maintain the natural environmental resource base has been a recurring cause of societal collapse (Diamond, 2004). Overuse and degradation of fresh-water supplies has been a particularly important problem. A well-known example is Easter Island in the southeast Pacific. The Polynesian people, who settled on the previously uninhabited island around 900 AD, initially thrived. However, they eventually denuded the island's forest, which led to massive soil erosion, loss of wood for canoes for fishing, and the extinction of pollinating birds. Their numbers dwindled, conditions deteriorated, and warfare and cannibalism broke out. When Dutch explorers landed in 1722, there were less than 2,000 inhabitants. By circa 1850, the survivors had dwindled to a few hundred.

Much earlier, the Mesopotamian civilizations in the Tigris-Euphrates valley had suffered from excessively intense agriculture and irrigation. Archaeological and historical evidence indicates that Sumeria, in the south, suffered from salinization of agricultural lands following extensive deforestation and irrigation (McMichael, 1993). Between 4,000 and 5,000 years ago, wheat was gradually replaced by barley, a more salt-tolerant cereal. During the subsequent half-millennium, Sumeria's agricultural productivity fell below the population's needs, political power receded, and the centre of that civilization migrated northwards to Babylon.

The Mayan civilization appears to have collapsed, around 1,000 years ago, under the dual stress of an adverse climatic cycle over several centuries and excessive agricultural demand on fresh water supplies. However, there is little evidence that environmental deterioration influenced the fall of the Greek, Roman, Inca or Ming Chinese civilizations.

Contemporary global environmental change

During the past two centuries, human impact on the environment has increased dramatically. Populations expanded approximately eight-fold and material-intensity and energy-intensity of economic activity greatly increased. World population, currently 6.3 billion, is expected to reach 8.5–9 billion by 2050. The total human 'carrying capacity' of Earth is uncertain, and depends on future patterns of consumption and waste generation. Today, we face unfamiliar problems posed by GEC. The best known is global climate change, occurring in response to the excessive emission of greenhouse gases into the lower atmosphere, especially the release of carbon dioxide from fossil fuel combustion. Figure 10.1 summarizes recent trends in average world temperature, and the authoritative estimated range of human-induced warming over the coming century (IPCC, 2001).

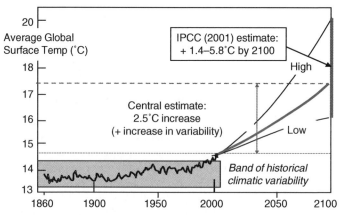

Figure 10.1 Time trends in average global surface temperature, and IPCC forecast for this century

Other GECs include:

* human-induced changes to the middle atmosphere and, therefore, function

    greenhouse gas accumulation, leading to climate change
    stratospheric ozone depletion;

* changes to global elemental cycles (nitrogen, phosphorus, sulphur, carbon, etc);
* biodiversity changes

    loss/extinction of species
    redistribution of species (invasion);

- changes to food-producing ecosystems;

    land cover, loss of soil fertility
    coastal and marine ecosystems (including fisheries);

- desertification;
- changes to the hydrological cycle, and depletion of freshwater supplies including major underground aquifers;
- worldwide dissemination of persistent organic pollutants (POPs);
- urbanization (e.g. land-use, pressure on regional ecosystems, massive waste generation).

Human alteration of Earth is substantial and growing. Between one-third and one-half of the land surface has been transformed by human action; the carbon dioxide concentration in the atmosphere has increased by nearly 30% since the beginning of the Industrial Revolution; more atmospheric nitrogen is fixed by humanity than by all natural terrestrial sources combined; more than half of all accessible surface fresh water is put to use by humanity; and about one-quarter of the bird species on Earth have been driven to extinction. By these and other standards, it is clear that we live on a human-dominated planet (Vitousek et al., 1997).

To understand better the systemic nature of these environmental changes, consider the world's carbon cycle. Carbon, the basis of life on Earth, circulates continuously between air, vegetation, soil and oceans. Meanwhile, vast and essentially immobile stores of carbon sit underground in ancient fossilized deposits of coal, oil and methane gas, and under the oceans as limestone sediment. Alongside the several hundred billion tonnes of carbon that circulate naturally through the biosphere each year, humans now annually release an extra 7–8 billion tonnes, primarily via fossil fuel combustion and forest clearance (an average of 1.3 tonnes of excess carbon per person annually). This distribution is very uneven: Americans, Australians and Canadians each contribute around 7 tonnes per year, while Africans and South Asians contribute less than a tonne. Some of this extra carbon is absorbed by Earth's natural 'sinks' (forests and oceans). However, the rest (approximately 3 billion tonnes) accumulates in the lower atmosphere as extra carbon dioxide which changes the heat-trapping capacity of the lower atmosphere, warming the Earth's surface. Without the natural 'greenhouse effect' of carbon dioxide and several other trace gases, Earth would be approximately 23°C colder (frozen!).

Relationship of global environmental changes to globalization

Globalization reflects the scale and connectedness of our economic, technological, cultural and other activities. At first sight, there seems to be a close connection between globalization and large-scale environmental change. After all, as industrialization spreads, the emission of greenhouse gases increases. Yet we seek a 'sustainable' future world, which will presumably be a globalized world (McMichael, 2002). This implies that globalization and GEC are not inextricably bound together.

Figure 10.2 shows the relationships between human populations and their economic and social activities, and the resultant changes in environmental stocks and conditions.

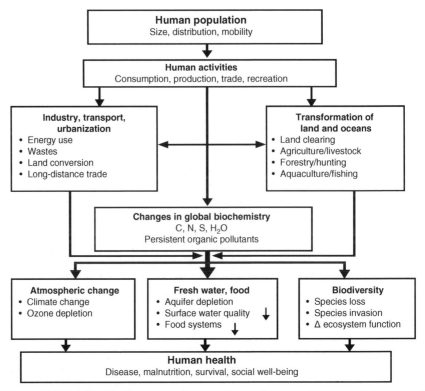

Figure 10.2 Relationships between societal activities, environmental impacts and changes, and resultant influences on human health

 Activity 10.1

1 List four ways (excluding the above-mentioned examples) in which globalization is likely to contribute to the occurrence of global (or at least internationally widespread) environmental change.

2 Name six key changes in technology or human practice that would render a future globalized world more ecologically sustainable.

 Feedback

1 Globalization might contribute to GEC in the following ways:

• Long-distance and rapid trade accelerates the inadvertent global distribution of 'exotic' species of insects, animals and plants. Some thrive in their new environments, disrupting ecosystems and displacing local food species.

• The intensification and increased corporate-control of world food production entails increasing use of energy and nitrogenous fertilizer. This has hugely increased the entry of activated nitrogenous compounds into the environment, changing the global nitrogen cycle, and causing significantly altered chemical balance and acidity in waterways and soils.

- The westernization of diets (in conjunction with rapid urbanization) stimulates demand for (excessive) meat consumption. This entails inefficient use of cereal grain as animal feed, and exerts great physical and chemical pressures on land and water resources. This includes deforestation to open up pastoral land. Widespread environmental degradation and carbon dioxide emissions result.
- As trade intensifies and spreads, many countries are driven to develop exports to generate foreign exchange. In exploiting their distinctive export opportunities, they may do so in ways that damage the local natural resource base. The widespread occurrence of uncontrolled logging is a well-known example, leading to widespread loss of locally valued forest products, species extinctions, flood control, mobilization of infectious agents (especially viruses) into human communities, and release of greenhouse gases.

2 Examples of technological and behavioural changes facilitating 'sustainability' are:

- De-carbonizing our energy generation (e.g. use of renewables such as wind power, nuclear energy, development of 'clean coal' technology).
- Reducing energy demands via public transport, energy-efficient domestic products, improved housing design.
- Laws that require imported (especially luxury) foods to reflect their full environmental cost (e.g. exhaust gases from air-freighted wine and foods).
- Re-orienting diets towards naturally health-promoting and environmentally benign production sources: fresh fruit and vegetables, meat in moderation (and produced by less fat-intensive means), unrefined carbohydrate foods.
- More rational use of antibiotics (limiting use in animal husbandry, houseplant cultivation, prescribing in humans) to retain some capacity to counter infectious disease agents.
- Re-engineering industry, agriculture and domestic/garden design to lessen the demand for fresh water; better technologies for the recycling of water.
- Controlled use of pesticides and herbicides, to minimize the (often long-term) damage to ecosystems and threatened extinction of species.

The risks to human health from GEC

The scale of GEC represents an important difference from environmental concerns that relate to localized toxicological or microbiological hazards. Indeed, these changes are manifestations of the 'ecological deficit' humans are forcing the planet into. Humans are crossing a new frontier, and there is a need to understand the range of likely adverse health impacts and other consequences (McMichael, 2001).

Before you consider the health risks of global climate change, a summary of the main known or anticipated health risks from other major categories of GEC is provided.

Stratospheric ozone depletion

Various human-produced industrial gases, especially halogenated compounds (such as the chlorofluorocarbons used for refrigeration and insulated packaging), destroy ozone molecules in the stratosphere. This allows greater penetration to the Earth's surface of solar ultraviolet radiation (UVR), particularly at higher (above approximately 35°) latitudes, including southern Australia, southern South America, Northern Europe and Canada. This increase in UVR exposure, particularly shorter-wavelength UV-B, increases the risk of skin cancer (malignant melanoma, non-melanocytic cancers). Other risks include increases in the incidence of ocular cataracts, other eye disorders such as squamous-cell cancer of the conjunctiva, and suppression of the immune system (e.g. lower vaccination efficacy, reduced risk of autoimmune disorders).

Disruption and degradation of various ecosystems

A major international scientific assessment of the current and estimated future conditions of the world's ecosystems, known as the Millennium Ecosystem Assessment Project, was carried out during 2001–04. It includes an assessment, by epidemiologists and others, of the consequences for human health. The increasing human demand for space, materials and food leads to increasingly rapid extinction of populations and species of plants and animals. This, in turn, can disrupt ecosystems that provide nature's goods and services. We may also lose, before discovery, many natural chemicals and genes with potential medical and health benefits. Myers (1997) estimates that five-sixths of the tropical vegetation useful for medicinal goods has not yet been recruited. Meanwhile, 'invasive' species are spreading into new environments in association with intensified trade, population mobility and food production. These bio-invasions have myriad consequences for health. For example, the spread of the water hyacinth in east Africa's Lake Victoria, introduced from Brazil as a decorative plant, has nurtured the water snails that transmit schistosomiasis and the proliferation of diarrhoeal disease organisms.

Impairment of food producing ecosystems

Increasing pressures from agricultural and livestock production put stresses on arable lands and pastures. In the early twenty-first century, an estimated one-third of the world's previously productive land is seriously damaged by erosion, compaction, salinization, waterlogging and chemicalization that destroy organic content. Similar pressures on the world's ocean fisheries have left most severely depleted or stressed. There is also doubt whether there is an environmentally benign and socially acceptable way of using genetic engineering to increase food yields. Such yields are needed to produce sufficient food for another 3 billion persons over the next half century.

Other global environmental changes

Freshwater supplies are coming under increasing pressure around the world. Various major (subterranean) aquifers, in all continents, are being depleted. Agricultural and industrial demand, amplified by population growth, often greatly exceeds both the rate of natural recharge of aquifers and flow rate within river systems. Water-related political crises and even open conflict seem likely to occur in the near future.

A number of semi-volatile persistent organic pollutants (POPs), such as poly-chlorinated biphenyls, are now disseminated worldwide. This occurs via a sequential distillation process across the adjoining 'cells' of the lower atmosphere at increasing latitudes, thereby transferring chemicals from their usual origins in low to mid latitudes, to high latitudes. Consequently, increasingly high levels of POPs are now being found in polar mammals and fish, as well as the human populations that traditionally eat them. Chemical pollution is no longer just an issue of local toxicity.

How do global environmental changes affect human health?

There are several pathways by which GEC can affect health. Figure 10.3 illustrates three pathways of increasingly more complex and less direct character. At the top, there are examples of how changes in basic physical environmental conditions (e.g. temperature extremes or level of ultraviolet irradiation) can affect human biology and health directly. The other two pathways illustrate processes

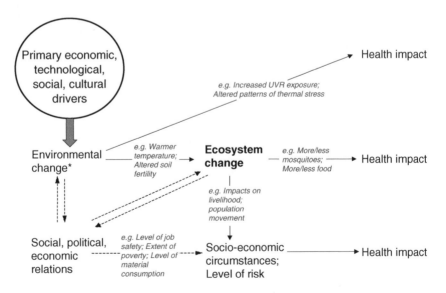

* e.g. climate change, ozone depletion, aquifer depletion, forest clearance, irrigation

Figure 10.3 Main pathways by which global environmental changes can affect human population health. The italicized items (on arrows) are illustrative only

of increasing complexity, including those that entail interactions between environmental conditions, ecosystem functioning, and human social and economic conditions.

 Activity 10.2

Fill in Table 10.1 (which shows nine types of GEC by eight categories of health risks) to indicate the known/likely strength of influence of each GEC on each health risk.

Use symbols to indicate very strong (++), somewhat strong (+), possible (?), and no influence (0). If you think that climate change has a strong influence on the risk of vector-borne infectious diseases, put a ++ in that cell as shown below.

 Feedback

Your response should look like Table 10.2.

Sustainability, health and well-being

There is growing discussion of the need to achieve sustainable environmental and social conditions. Achieving sustainability means not passing critical thresholds that would cause irreversible and detrimental changes such as the permanent collapse of major fisheries, melting of large polar ice-sheets (raising sea-levels several metres), or collapse of a state due to social disorder and violence. In other words, sustainability is about maintaining the ecological systems and processes upon which healthy life depends. Relatedly, the attainment of what has been called a balanced 'triple bottom line' (i.e. optimizing economic, social and environmental conditions) should be seen as a *means*, not an *end*. The rationale for a high-grade 'triple bottom-line' is to enhance human experience, including health and survival.

Long-term optimization of human experience is the true bottom-line of 'sustainability', with health as a central criterion. Sustainability will require us to achieve societies able to maintain the natural resource base, and its ecosystems, and to maintain internal social cohesion. As noted earlier, humankind is now over-loading the biosphere. This is illustrated in Figure 10.4 based on the systematic estimation of our collective 'ecological footprint' (Wackernagel et al., 2002). The ecological footprint is an accounting term for ecological resources, developed by the Task Force on Health and Sustainable Communities at the University of British Columbia. It corresponds to the area of productive land and aquatic ecosystems required to produce the resources used and to assimilate the wastes produced by a defined population at a specified material standard of living, wherever on Earth that land may be located.

Table 10.1 Influence of nine types of GEC on eight health risks

	Physical injuries	Mental health impacts	Hunger and malnutrition	Infectious disease: VBDs	Infectious disease: Water- and food-borne	Cancers	Respiratory diseases	Cardio-vascular (heart blood vessels) diseases
Climate change				‡				
Ozone depletion, and UVR exposure								
Disruption of elemental cycles								
Freshwater depletion								
Soil degradation								
Biodiversity loss								
Damage to marine and coastal ecosystems								
Persistent organic pollutants (POPs)								
Urbanization and its impacts								

Table 10.2 Influence of nine types of GEC on eight health states (completed)

	Physical injuries	Mental health impacts	Hunger and malnutrition	Infectious disease: VBDs	Infectious disease: Water- and food-borne	Cancers	Respiratory diseases	Cardio-vascular (heart blood vessels) diseases
Climate change	‡	+	+	‡	‡	?	+	+
Ozone depletion, and UVR exposure	0	0	0	?	?	‡	0	0
Disruption of elemental cycles	0	+	?	0	0	0	0	0
Freshwater depletion	0	?	+	0	‡	0	0	0
Soil degradation	0	?	‡	0	0	+	0	?
Biodiversity loss	0	0	‡	0	0	0	0	0
Damage to marine and coastal ecosystems	0	0	?	0	0	+	+	0
Persistent organic pollutants (POPs)	0	0	0	0	0	?	?	0
Urbanization and its impacts	+	+	0	+	+	?	?	?

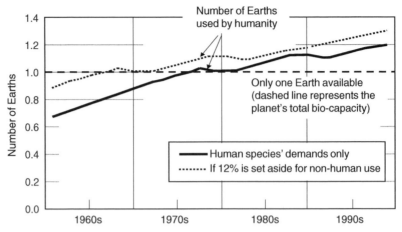

Based on Wackernagel et al., 2002.

Figure 10.4 Estimates of the human overloading of the biocapacity of the Earth

Note: The figures are indicative only. It appears that we have been operating in ecological deficit over the past quarter-century.

 Activity 10.3

If you have access to the Internet, go to one (or both) of the two *Ecological Footprint* websites below. If you do a web search on 'ecological footprint' you will find similar personal footprint estimating sites. Estimate your personal footprint size.

 Feedback

Your footprint size is about ten minutes. The result tells you how many Earths would be needed if all 6.4 billion humans had a lifestyle like yours.

1 http://www.lead.org/leadnet/footprint/intro.htm

This simple questionnaire calculates a relatively accurate Ecological Footprint for an individual living in the US (the default answers represent North American averages). The 13 questions cover food, transportation and housing. The application then calculates your Ecological Footprint. For a more detailed analysis of individual ecological footprints, or to learn more about the Ecological Footprint methodology and applications, contact Redefining Progress at http://www.rprogress.org.

2 http://www.earthday.org/footprint/index.asp (widely accessible without broadband)

How much of 'nature' does your lifestyle require? This Ecological Footprint Quiz estimates how much productive land and water you need to support what you use and discard. By answering 15 questions, you can compare your footprint to others, and to what is available on this planet.

Global climate change and health

The climate system and greenhouse gases

To date the most extensive, and best developed, GEC-related health risk assessments have been done in relation to stratospheric ozone depletion (with its mostly direct-acting risks to skin and eyes) and global climate change. This section focuses on the latter, as exemplar of global environmental change, and examines the methods of studying, and estimating, the resultant health impacts.

There remains debate about the relationship between human-generated 'greenhouse gases' and the world's climate system. Over the past decade, the number of doubters has declined steadily as the science of climate change has matured, and some early signs of the (non-human) impact of recent global warming have begun to appear. Several things are known as facts:

1 Various greenhouse gases (GHG), especially carbon dioxide and water vapour, occur naturally in the atmosphere. By capturing some of the solar energy re-radiated outwards by Earth, those GHG warm the Earth's surface by around 32°C. The physics of this process is well understood.
2 Over aeons the atmospheric concentration of GHG has varied in close correlation with the temperature of the Earth's surface.
3 Other factors affect the Earth's temperature, including variation in solar activity; the amount of volcanic activity; and (on longer time-scales) the tilt of the Earth's axis and shape of its orbit.

Given this scientific knowledge, and that GHG concentration has risen 35% since the beginning of the Industrial Revolution 200 years ago, scientists predict that the Earth's temperature will rise. It has in fact risen unusually fast over the past quarter-century, and the temporal and spatial characteristics of this rise indicate that most has been due to the increasing concentration of GHG. Nevertheless, uncertainties remain about the future GHG-emitting behaviours of societies, how the complex climate system will respond to future changes in atmospheric composition, how feedback processes will operate, and whether there are critical thresholds that will cause abrupt climatic-environmental changes. Vigorous debate therefore continues about the projected actual trajectories of global temperature over the coming century.

There are five layers of atmosphere. The lowest layer (troposphere), where 'weather' occurs, extends 8–16 kilometres. On average, temperature in the troposphere decreases by 7°C for each kilometre increase in altitude. At the top of the troposphere, temperatures can be as low as −58°C. The next layer (stratosphere) extends to about 50 kilometre altitude, with temperatures slowly *increasing* to about 4°C at the top. The high concentration of ozone that occurs naturally at around 20–25 kilometre altitude absorbs most of the sun's ultraviolet rays. Next there are three more layers (mesosphere, thermosphere and exosphere) characterized by falling, then rising, temperature patterns.

Naturally-occurring greenhouse gases (including water vapour, carbon dioxide, nitrous oxide, methane and ozone) comprise about 2% of the atmosphere. The Earth's surface absorbs some solar radiation and reradiates it outwards as long-wave (infrared) radiation. Some of this infrared radiation is absorbed by atmospheric greenhouse gases and reradiated back to Earth, thus raising the average surface temperature to its present 15°C. Without this warming, the average temperature of the Earth would be about 33°C colder and permanently frozen over.

World average temperature and atmospheric carbon dioxide concentration has varied over the past 420,000 years. These have been estimated from the chemistry of the annually-layered Antarctic ice cores. Earth's temperature has naturally varied within a range of 10°C, as the planet has moved in and out of global glaciations. It is against this background that humankind is now superimposing additional carbon dioxide 'greenhouse forcing'. Indeed, the concentration of carbon dioxide has reached 380 parts per million (ppm) in 2004, an almost 40% increase on the pre-industrial 275 ppm. Most of the recent emissions have occurred during the twentieth century as a result of burgeoning economic activity. Currently, the rate of emission remains unabated as industrialization proceeds in the developing world. China, India and Brazil are now becoming major emitters.

In its Third Assessment Report, the UN's Intergovernmental Panel on Climate Change stated: 'There is new and stronger evidence that most of the warming observed over the last 50 years is attributable to human activities' (IPCC, 2001). During the twentieth century, world average surface temperature increased by approximately 0.6°C (Figure 10.1), and two-thirds of that warming occurred after 1975. As shown in Figures 10.1 and 10.8, the IPPC forecasts a rise in average world temperature of around 3–4°C over the coming century, although there is still some uncertainty around this estimate. The warming would be greater at higher latitudes, on land than at sea, and would affect night-time more than day-time temperatures. Alaska, northern Canada and northern Siberia are likely to warm by approximately 5°C this century. This anticipated warming would be much more rapid than any natural warming experienced by humans since the advent of agriculture around 10,000 years ago. This extremely rapid rate of change will put many of the biosphere's ecosystems and species under stress.

There would also be regional changes in rainfall patterns, with increases over the oceans but reduction over much of the land surface, especially in various low-to-medium latitude mid-continental regions (central Spain, US midwest, Sahel, Amazonia), and in already arid areas in northwest India, the Middle East, northern Africa and parts of Central America. Rainfall events would tend to intensify, with more frequent extreme events increasing the likelihood of flooding and droughts. Regional weather systems, including the great South-West Asian monsoon, could undergo latitudinal shift.

Climatologists also anticipate that climate variability will increase with global climate change. Computer models and empirical evidence suggest there will be increasingly severe weather events including more powerful storms and stronger winds, intensification of the El Niño cycle, and altered patterns of drought and rainfall. There is great inertia in the climate system. Even if the build-up in greenhouse gases is arrested by mid-century, the seas would continue to expand as the extra heat permeates the oceans, rising by up to several metres over the coming thousand years. There is a small possibility that parts of the Antarctic ice mass would melt, immediately raising sea-level by several metres.

Another possibility (depicted, with some licence, in the film *The Day After Tomorrow)* is that the northern Atlantic Gulf Stream might weaken, and eventually

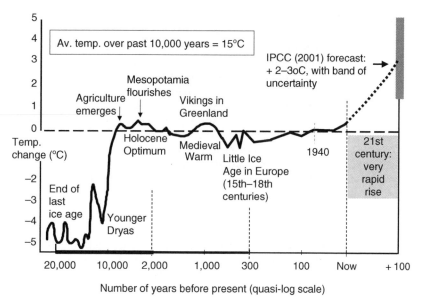

Figure 10.5 Variations in Earth's average surface temperature, over the past 20,000 years
Source: McMichael (1993).

shut down, as increased melt-water from the Greenland glacier disrupts the great, slow 'conveyor belt' circulation that distributes Pacific-equatorial warm water around the world's oceans. Northwestern Europe, relative to same-latitude Newfoundland, currently enjoys 5–7°C of free heating from this source. If the Gulf Stream weakens over the coming century or two, Europe may actually become colder even as the rest of the world warms.

With two-thirds of the world's population living within 60 kilometres of the sea, a rise in sea-level would have widespread health impacts. The countries most vulnerable to sea-level rise include Bangladesh and Egypt, with huge river delta farming populations, and Pakistan, Indonesia and Thailand, with large coastal populations. Various low-lying small-island populations in the Pacific and Indian Oceans, with few material resources, face the prospect of wholesale displacement. A half-metre rise would approximately double the number (at today's population) who experience flooding annually from around 50 million to 100 million. Some of the world's coastal arable land and fish-nurturing mangroves would be damaged by sea-level rise. Rising seas would salinate coastal freshwater aquifers, particularly under small islands. A heightening of storm surges would damage coastal roadways, sanitation systems and housing.

Over the coming century, as shown earlier in Figure 10.1, world average temperature is predicted to increase 1.4–5.8°C. This anticipated increase will be greater at higher latitudes, and winter than in summer.

Health impacts of climate change

There are direct and indirect ways in which climate change can affect human health. Further, some impacts will occur relatively immediately, while others will depend on a succession of changes in natural systems, and may occur incrementally. Figure 10.6 summarizes these various pathways and should be regarded as indicative, not comprehensive. It should also be noted that there is, as yet, little empirical evidence that the process of climate *change* causes these health impacts. The anticipation and estimation of these health risks depends on extrapolation from the climate-health relationships previously observed within situations of natural climate variation and local trend. Hence, there is some debate as to when and where health impacts attributable to climate change *per se* might actually occur.

The anticipated direct health impacts include those due to changes in exposure to thermal extremes (heat and cold); increases in extreme weather events (floods, cyclones, storm-surges, droughts); and increased production of certain air pollutants and aeroallergens (spores and moulds). Decreases in winter mortality due to milder winters may compensate for increases in summer mortality due to the increased frequency of heatwaves.

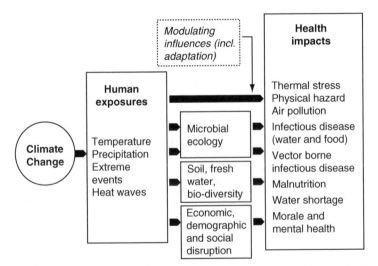

Figure 10.6 Pathways, direct and indirect, by which climate change affects human health

Climate change, acting via less direct mechanisms, would affect regional food productivity. It would affect the transmission of many infectious diseases, especially water-, food- and vector-borne diseases. Recent reports suggest that we may now be seeing some early impacts of climate change on infectious diseases. For example, tick-borne (viral) encephalitis in Sweden appears to have increased in response to a succession of warmer winters over the past two decades, and there is some (contentious) evidence of malaria ascending to higher altitudes in the eastern African highlands in association with local warming (Patz et al., 2002). In the longer term, these indirect impacts are likely to have greater magnitude than more direct impacts.

Vector-borne infections are of particular relevance. The distribution and abundance of vector organisms and intermediate hosts are affected by physical factors (temperature, precipitation, humidity, surface water and wind) and biotic factors (vegetation, host species, predators, parasites and human interventions). Modelling studies indicate that a temperature increase would cause net increases, worldwide, in the geographic range of various vector organisms, although some localized decreases might occur. Further, temperature-related changes in the life cycle of both vector and pathogen (flukes, protozoa, bacteria and viruses) would increase the potential transmission of many vector-borne diseases: malaria (mosquito), dengue (mosquito) and leishmaniasis (sand-fly), although schisto-somiasis (water-snail) may undergo a net decrease (if water temperatures in many regions become too warm for the snail to thrive).

The mathematical models used to make such projections have well-recognized limitations, but their use has provided an important first-order understanding. For example, from a series of modelling studies it seems likely that malaria will significantly extend its geographic range of *potential* transmission, and its seasonality, during the twenty-first century as average temperatures rise (Martens et al., 1999). Figure 10.7 illustrates the modelling of the impact of forecast changes in temperature and rainfall in Australia on the geographic range of the mosquito species that transmits viral dengue fever.

Modelling, allowing for future trends in trade and economic development, has been used to estimate the impacts of climate change on cereal grain yields (which account for 50–60% of world food energy). The results indicate that a slight downturn is likely over the next half-century, but this would be greater in already food-insecure regions in South Asia, parts of Africa and Central America. Such downturns would increase the number of malnourished people by several tens of millions in the world, against a current and projected total without climate change of between 800 million and 400 million, respectively.

Of course, the health prospects are not all negative. Milder winters would reduce the seasonal winter-time mortality peak in temperate countries. A further increase in temperatures in currently hot regions might impair mosquito survival. Overall, however, scientists have consistently assessed that most climate change health impacts would be adverse (IPCC, 2001).

As average surface temperatures gradually rise, an increase in climatic variability is likely. Indeed, the frequency and intensity of such events already appears to be increasing. Many scientists consider that human health and safety are more endangered by an impending increase in extreme and anomalous weather events than by changes in average climate conditions. The following extract by Johnathon Patz (2004) describes the possibilities of abrupt changes in health risks.

Global warming

Health impacts may be abrupt as well as long term

The doomsday film thriller *The Day After Tomorrow* is based on global warming theory, whereby the infusion of freshwater into the north Atlantic from the melting of Greenland's glaciers stops the circulation of water via the Gulf Stream. Although the probability of this event is low, according to climatologists, the scenario of abrupt climate change has certainly caught Hollywood's imagination.

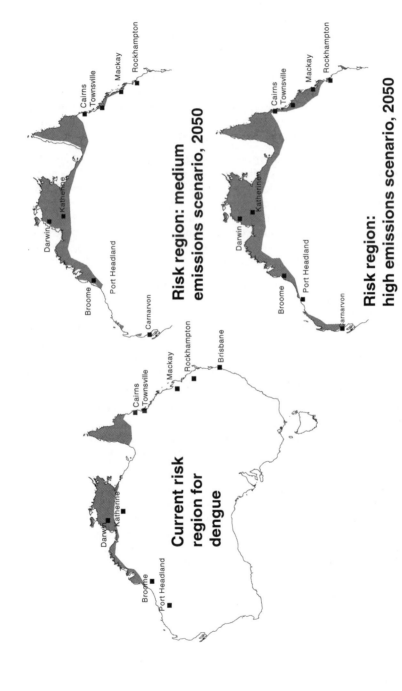

Figure 10.7 Estimated 'risk region' for maintaining dengue mosquito vector at present and under alternative future climate scenarios in 2050

Source: McMichael (2003).

Not surprisingly, the prospect of extreme weather events also has caught the real concern of health experts (not just their imaginations), following on the heels of last year's devastating heat wave, as a result of which an estimated 15 000 people in France died in a matter of a weeks. The extent to which the severity of the European heat wave falls far outside the current distribution of weather is consistent with expectations of future climate change scenarios. Climatologists have long remarked that global warming will not simply manifest itself by a gradual climb in average temperatures. Rather, it is the frequency and intensity of extreme climatic events – such as heat waves, droughts, floods, and storms – that are expected to occur.

Extreme weather events such as severe storms, floods, and drought have claimed millions of lives during the past 20 years and have adversely affected the lives of many more as well as costing enormous amounts in property damage. On average, the number of people killed annually by weather disasters between 1972 and 1996 was about 123 000, most of them in Africa and Asia. For every one person killed in a natural disaster, 1000 people are affected, either physically or through loss of property or livelihood.

River floods in central Europe left over 200 000 people homeless; more than 100 people were killed, and due to climate change such floods are projected to increase. Degradation of the local environment can also contribute to vulnerability from flooding. For example, Hurricane Mitch, the most deadly hurricane to strike the western hemisphere in the past two centuries, caused 11 000 deaths and thousands of others were missing in Central America. Many fatalities occurred as a result of mudslides in deforested areas.

Studies of the effect of climate change on food production show that yields of cereal grains are likely to decrease in the tropics where many countries are already under water stress. In particular there is concern that climate change may increase the extent of malnutrition in Africa, and there is currently widespread evidence of under-nutrition in countries of central, southern, and eastern Africa. Drought also leads to forest fires, which in some locations (especially Malaysia and Brazil) have been associated with an increased risk of respiratory disease, eye problems, injuries, and fatalities.

The El Niño phenomenon is the strongest short term driver of climate variability worldwide (excluding seasonal variability). It already causes natural disasters that pose health risks, particularly droughts, on a global scale. The difference in numbers of people affected by disasters between a pre-El Niño and post-El Niño a year is on average around 2.7% of the world's population. A large number of case reports and a smaller number of time series analyses over more than one event show a range of impacts of El Niño on health. The most consistent associations are with malaria epidemics in parts of Latin America and South Asia, but outbreaks of cholera, hantavirus infection, Rift Valley fever, and other diseases have also been associated with El Niño. Although this is still being debated, more and more climatologists believe that global warming may increase the frequency and intensity of El Niño events: not good news for the health sector.

Although extreme weather variability affects injuries, fatalities, and the incidence of diseases such as malaria, we must not lose sight of the myriad of other diseases and health outcomes affected by more subtle long term climate change.

Mosquito borne diseases, such as dengue fever and encephalitis, are generally more influenced by ambient conditions than diseases passed directly from human to human. Formation of ozone air pollution is hastened by warmer temperatures. Excessive rainfall and runoff can lead to large numbers of microorganisms entering drinking water, and outbreaks of waterborne disease have been associated with heavy rainfall events in the United States and elsewhere.

Although the doomsday scenarios may be far from reality, the slower march of climate change still presents a formidable challenge for the health sector and society as a whole. A tidal wave inundating a city is an easily identifiable disaster that, given enough warning, people may escape from. The many health effects posed by climate change will arrive through numerous convoluted pathways and will require interdisciplinary analyses and integrated prevention planning.

 Activity 10.4

1 What climate-related health events can you think of within the past 12 months, in your region of the world or elsewhere, that might illustrate the possibility of rapid changes in risks to health, or of 'surprise' impacts?
2 How easy/reasonable is it, at this stage, to attribute any such individual impact event to human-induced climate change?

 Feedback

1 An example is the extreme heatwave of August 2003 in Europe that increased mortality significantly in some countries.

2 It's difficult, which is why more research and monitoring is required.

Estimating current and future burdens of disease attributable to climate change

To relate estimates of health risks more directly to policy and social decision making, it is desirable to estimate the plausible range of future burdens of health impacts attributable to climate change. This can be done globally, regionally, nationally or locally. WHO's *World Health Report 2002* estimates that, by 2000, global climate change was already responsible for 2.4% of diarrhoeal disease worldwide, and up to 6–7% of malaria and dengue in specified groups of countries. These figures were based on a wide-ranging international study that used standardized methods to quantify and compare the population burdens of diverse health outcomes (Ezzati et al., 2004).

Summary

You have learnt how the impact of global environmental changes are complex. Scientific opinion points clearly to an urgent need to address the sustainability of global changes currently taking place. While public health research to identify current and future health risks from GEC remains challenging, research on the health impacts of climate change has already yielded key insights.

References

Ezzati M, Lopez A, Rodgers A and Murray C, eds (2004) *Comparative quantification of health risks: global and regional burden of disease attributable to selected major risk factors.* Geneva: WHO.

Intergovernmental Panel on Climate Change (IPCC) (2001) *Climate Change 2001. The Third Assessment Report* (3 volumes). New York: Cambridge University Press.

Martens W et al. (1999) 'Climate change and future populations at risk of malaria.' *Global Environmental Change* 9 Suppl: S89–107.

McMichael AJ (1993) *Planetary Overload: Global Environmental Change and the Health of the Human Species.* Cambridge: Cambridge University Press.

McMichael AJ (2001) *Human frontiers, environments and disease: past patterns, uncertain futures.* Cambridge: Cambridge University Press.

McMichael AJ, Woodruff R, Whetton P, Hennessy K, et al. (2003) *Human Health and Climate Change in Oceania: A Risk Assessment.* Canberra: Commonwealth Government, p. 126.

Myers N (1997) 'Biodiversity's genetic library.' In *Nature's Services. Societal Dependence on Natural Ecosystems* (Myers N, ed.). Washington, DC: Island Press, 255–73.

Patz JA (2004) 'Global Warming – health impacts may be abrupt as well as long term.' *BMJ*, 328: 1269–70.

Patz JA, Hulme M, Rosenzweig C, Mitchell TD, Goldberg RA, Githeko AK, Lele S, Anthony J, McMichael AJ and Le Sueur D (2002) 'Increasing incidence of malaria since 1970 parallels regional warming in East Africa.' *Nature*, 420: 627–8.

WHO (2003) *World Health Report 2002.* Geneva: WHO.

Global health and security

Overview

In this chapter you will examine the linking of global health issues with the field of security. You will begin with an introduction to the concept of security, and the key debates surrounding how security is defined before examining the links between global health and security by examining the specific examples of bioterrorism, emerging and re-emerging infectious diseases and HIV/AIDS.

Learning objectives

After working through this chapter, you will be able to:

- **define the concepts of national and human security**
- **review trends towards a broadening of the security agenda**
- **identify three criteria for defining global health issues as security issues**
- **recognize why biological weapons, emerging and re-emerging infectious diseases, and HIV/AIDS are receiving increasing attention from the security community**
- **understand the benefits and risks of linking global health with a security agenda.**

Key terms

Global health security The set of issues where global health and national security concerns overlap, including infectious disease epidemics and bioterrorism.

Human security The protection of individual life and well-being from threats.

National security The defence of the state against military and other types of serious threats to the state's survival and well-being.

How can security be defined?

Security is a contested concept. Scholars of security studies and practitioners within the security policy community have offered dozens of definitions over the past 60 years, with none achieving the widespread recognition of, for example, the definition of health within the World Health Organization (WHO) Constitution.

Disagreement covers all aspects of the term 'security' save one: that security entails freedom from threat or danger.

Whose security, whether that of individuals, communities or states, is the central question within ongoing debates. Disputes about the object of security, in turn, give rise to questions about the nature of potential threats. These can range from traditional military threats, to a broader view that include threats to ecological and day-to-day well-being. You can consider the questions of whose security and type of security threat by considering the following definition by Lippman (1943):

> 'A nation [state] is secure to the extent to which it is not in danger of having to sacrifice core values if it wishes to avoid war, and is able, if challenged, to maintain them by victory in such a war.'

In this definition, Lippman places the interests of the nation-state as the primary object of security. In other words it is the protection of the nation-state, and promotion of its vital interests, that lies at the heart of this definition.

There are three alternative ways of thinking about the object of security. First, you might define security 'below the state'; that is, in terms of the security of an individual or community of people within a state. For example, the concept of human security focuses on the security needs of individual persons. Second, you might define security 'across the state' when security concerns a community of people who live across a number of states. The Kurdish or Roma people, for example, are not strictly defined by a state identity. Third, security can be defined 'above the state' when the focus is the security of a group of states, a region or even the global community as a whole. For example, strategic alliances such as the North Atlantic Treaty Organization (NATO) and former Warsaw Pact (of the Soviet Union and eastern European allies) seek to protect the collective security of certain states. The concept of global environmental security focuses above, and even beyond, the state by seeking to protect the integrity of large scale biosystems that enable life on Earth.

As well as understanding the object of security, it is also important to define what factors are seen to potentially threaten security. The second part of Lippman's definition focuses on war, and by implication, on military threats. His definition is not easily extended to threats that are non-military in nature. For example, an economic crisis, such as a sudden and significant currency devaluation, an environmental threat like global warming, or a health threat like the outbreak of a lethal and highly contagious infectious disease would not typically require a state to go to war, and therefore not meet Lippman's definition of a security issue.

The questions of what is the object of security, and how security is defined, are critical. As Wolfers wrote in 1952, but which is equally true today, 'any reference to the pursuit of security is likely to ring a sympathetic chord'. While appearing to offer clearer direction to policy and action, the term 'security' remains ambiguous until further defined. He argues that the ambiguity of the term 'may be permitting everyone to label whatever policy he favours with an attractive and possibly deceptive name.'

In summary, there are two important aspects of security to consider. The first is the object of security, or whose security is important. The answer can be located at different levels, from the individual, to communities, to the state, to a collection of states, to the entire world. The second aspect of security is how a threat to security is defined. Traditionally, threats are seen as military in nature. However other types of threats exist, and can vary depending on the object of security identified. You will now consider two main levels of security in closer detail – the state and the individual.

National security

The traditional and still dominant approach to security studies focuses on national security, whereby each state sees the protection of its vital interests as the priority of its government. National security has traditionally been pursued as the number one priority of governments because, it is argued, without survival of the state, no other priorities or goals of government can be achieved. Governments seek to protect and promote their national security through their military, economic, domestic and foreign policies.

During the Cold War era, when tensions between the US and Soviet Union defined international relations, national security policies predominantly focused on external military threats. Governments sought to defend against such threats through the accumulation of military power and making of strategic alliances with other states. This perspective, known as the *realist* (or *realpolitik*) approach, assumes that international relations are defined by states competing for power. The nuclear arms race between the two superpowers is a clear example of both sides seeking to enhance their security by building up a formidable arsenal. The related concept of collective security is also focused on the national interests of states. However, it argues that states can cooperate, rather than compete, to create a more stable and peaceful international system.

Beginning in the early 1980s, but especially since the end of the Cold War, western governments sought to understand what new threats might now be faced. A proliferation of writing sought to broaden the concept of security by evaluating new non-military threats to security. While military and economic threats remain a core component of national security, other issues such as mass migrations, environmental degradation and acute epidemic infections are now considered possible threats to state security. Moreover, many of these 'new security threats' are transnational in character, where either the cause or effect may transcend national borders. These transnational threats pose new challenges for states seeking to secure national interests.

Human security

The rethinking of national security in the 1990s also led to development of the concept of human security. The human security perspective explicitly shifts the object of security from the state to the individual. The United Nations Development Programme (UNDP) *Human Development Report 1994* states,

'The concept of security has for too long been interpreted narrowly: as security of territory from external aggression, or a protection of national interests in foreign policy or as global security from the threat of nuclear holocaust . . . Forgotten were the legitimate concerns of ordinary people who sought security in their daily lives.'

Human security is defined as safety from such chronic threats as hunger, disease and repression. And second, it means protection from sudden and hurtful disruptions in the patterns of daily life – whether in homes, in jobs or in communities. As you see in this definition, human security is defined broadly to encompass a range of threats to the individual.

From this perspective, there is scepticism about the ability of the state to fully provide human security. Under certain circumstances, the state may even become the major source of insecurity for individuals. For example, for Jews and other minorities in Nazi Germany, and Tutsi in Rwanda in 1994, the state represented the primary human security threat. Instead of relying on the state, human security focuses on non-state actors and transnational social movements to protect and empower individuals.

Most supporters of human security recognize its interdependence with national security (Commission on Human Security, 2003). When a state is insecure, it is very difficult for individuals within that state to remain secure. Similarly, state security is built upon the security of its individual citizens. When individuals are insecure, it becomes more difficult for the basic functions of the state to operate. Despite the difficulties of separating national and human security in theory, in practice the national security perspective remains dominant, while the human security approach is largely confined within the development community.

Table 11.1 Perspectives on security

Concept	Basic focus	Security objective
National Security/Realism	Power politics among states	Security for the state
Collective security	The individual, democracy and interdependence	Security among states for the benefit of individuals
Human security	Structural injustice and transnationalism	Security for individuals and communities through transnational civil society action
Ecological security	Biological/environmental threats	Sustainable equilibrium between the natural environment, pathogens and human populations

Activity 11.1

Read the following two definitions of security. For each definition, describe who the object of security is and give three examples of a security threat defined in this way.

1 'A threat to national security is an action or sequence of events that (1) threatens drastically and over a relatively brief span of time to degrade the quality of life for inhabitants of a state, or (2) threatens significantly to narrow the range of policy choices available to the government of a state or to private, nongovernmental entities (persons, groups, corporations) within the state.' (Ullman, 1983)

2 'Human security means protecting fundamental freedoms – freedoms that are the essence of life. It means protecting people from critical and pervasive threats and situations. It means using processes that build on people's strengths and aspirations. It means creating political, social, environmental, economic, military and cultural systems that together give people the building blocks of survival, livelihood and dignity.' (Commission on Human Security, 2003)

 Feedback

For the first definition, the object of security is the state. Threats to the national security of a state might include a military attack, sudden flood of refugees due to a conflict in a neighbouring state or economic crisis. The object of security in the second definition is the individual. Threats to human security might include loss of employment, lack of basic needs such as food and water, or local environmental disaster.

How is health related to security?

The Commission on Human Security (2003) writes that 'good health is both essential and instrumental to achieving human security.' Good health is 'essential' because illness, disability and death are critical threats to human security. Good health is 'instrumental' because it allows people to exercise choice in their lives. The Commission argues that violence, infectious diseases and poverty are the three health challenges that critically impact human security (see Figure 11.1).

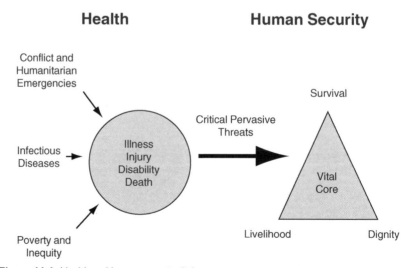

Figure 11.1 Health and human security linkages

Source: Is based on Commission on Human Security (2003).

Perhaps more surprising is how selected health issues have come to be included among the traditional concerns of national security. Health has traditionally been relegated to so-called 'low politics'; that is, a domestic concern of social policy unworthy of priority consideration at the 'top table' of 'high-politics' occupied by foreign, defence and economic policy. Describing the new engagement between health and national security, Nils Daulaire (2003), President and CEO of the Global Health Council, writes:

> 'Most of us in health professions have a simple response to the question of why we engage in global health: because it is right to help those who are sick and in need, and because this is at the heart of our calling ... But there exists an argument beyond the moral and humanitarian aspects of global health. In a changing and dangerous world, United States engagement in global health has emerged as a fundamental national interest.'

The concept of global health security is the area where national security and global health concerns overlap. The overlap between the two fields is limited and highly contested. Which issues are considered global health security issues is a critical question. The security community seeks to understand whether certain global health issues threaten core interests of the state. The global health community seeks higher-level political attention and funding for such health issues.

Clearly not all global health issues have been considered threats to national security. While no systematic criteria exist, examination of the issues discussed so far as security threats helps to identify what criteria have been used to define global health security concerns. To become part of a national security agenda, a global health issue is likely to:

- pose a severe risk to social well-being by impacting population health status, the health status of a strategic group such as the armed forces, or the economy;
- have an impact across borders and notably in strategically important countries; or
- pose an acute threat in a relatively immediate timeframe.

These criteria help to explain why some long-term health issues that cause high morbidity and mortality, such as chronic diseases, are not presently considered national security threats. Whose security is being considered is also an important determinant. While countries with HIV prevalence rates above 30% may consider the disease a security threat to their own survival, countries with lower prevalence may only consider the disease a security threat if its incidence in other countries create transborder consequences, such as high rates of imported infections.

To understand these criteria in more detail, and in relation to specific health issues, the following sections will examine bioterrorism, emerging and re-emerging infectious diseases, and HIV/AIDS.

Bioterrorism and biological weapons

> 'We have entered an era of catastrophic terrorism in which our greatest vulnerability will be created by our own technological sophistication – the phenomenon of blowback – in which the technology and infrastructure

that contribute to our economic comfort and social welfare can be exploited by terrorists determined to damage us, erode people's confidence in government, and provoke legislative actions that erode our civil liberties.' (Poste, 2002)

The spectre of biological weapons represents the clearest link between health and national security policy. Biological warfare (BW) is the deliberate spread of disease among an adversary's population, livestock or plant life. BW involves the use of living organisms or the by-products of living organisms as instruments for waging conflict. The development of biological weapons based on these diseases is attractive to states and terrorist organizations because they:

- have the potential to cause mass casualties;
- can be made with materials and information that are widely available and commonly used in legitimate commercial activities;
- are significantly less expensive to produce and easier to conceal than a comparable nuclear programme.

The intentional use of biological weapons by a state, group or individual fits easily into *realist* definitions of security that emphasize the defence of the state from external military threats. The terms biosecurity and biological security are used to describe attempts to protect a state against biological attack.

While the use of disease as a weapon of war dates back many centuries, three events during the mid-1990s brought biological weapons onto both the national security and global health agendas. In 1995, Iraqi defectors revealed a larger and more sophisticated biological weapons programme than previously known, including the production of *Bacillus anthracis* and the botulinum toxin (Henderson, 1998). The same year the Japanese Aum Shinrikyo cult attacked the Tokyo subway with Sarin gas. These events were followed by a series of revelations, following the end of the Cold War, about the extent of the former Soviet Union's biological weapons programmes. Indeed, the Soviet signing of the 1972 Biological and Toxin Weapons Convention was viewed as an opportunity to significantly expand the Soviet biological weapons programme. Similarly, the global eradication of smallpox in 1979 was secretly followed by a Soviet programme to produce and weaponize the smallpox virus. Realization that these programmes were more extensive than previously believed caused great concern within the international community (Henderson, 1998).

Following the attack on the World Trade Center in September 2001, five letters containing *Bacillus anthracis* were mailed to US government officials and media outlets. Twenty-two people developed anthrax, and five died, as a result. Despite the relatively low number of deaths, the incident caused massive disruption. Senate office buildings and postal facilities were closed, US mail irradiated, and 33,000 people required prophylaxis. These events led to large-scale efforts and collaboration between the public health and security communities to enhance domestic preparedness. The highest priority bioterrorism agents, according to the US Centers for Disease Control and Prevention are those that pose a risk to national security because they:

- can be easily disseminated or transmitted from person to person;
- result in high mortality rates and have the potential for major public health impact;

- might cause public panic and social disruption; and
- require special action for public health preparedness.

These agents are:

- anthrax (bacillus anthracis);
- botulism (clostridium botulinum toxin);
- plague (yersinia pestis);
- smallpox (variola major);
- tularemia (francisella tularensis);
- viral haemorrhagic fevers (filoviruses [e.g. ebola, marburg] and arenaviruses [e.g. lassa, machupo]).

To date the failure to prosecute the perpetrator of the anthrax attacks demonstrates the difficulty of attributing bioterrororist attacks to a particular state or non-state actor. The development and proliferation of biological weapons is a transnational problem, which poses a new challenge for both the health and security communities.

Emerging and re-emerging infectious diseases

'In the context of infectious diseases, there is nowhere in the world from which we are remote and no one from whom we are disconnected.' (US Institute of Medicine, 1992)

The last 30 years have witnessed the emergence of new diseases alongside the resurgence of old diseases, some increasingly resistant to antimicrobials and drug treatment. At least 30 new diseases have been identified since 1973, a rate of almost one per year. Previously known diseases such as cholera, yellow fever and dengue have re-emerged dramatically, and some like tuberculosis, have re-emerged in multi-drug resistant forms. Disease vectors have also become resistant to insecticides and increased their geographic range, bringing malaria, African sleeping sickness, West Nile virus, Rift Valley fever, yellow fever and dengue into new areas and onto new continents (as you saw in Chapter 5).

Emerging and re-emerging infectious diseases (ERIDs) were not generally viewed as threats to national security until the 1990s. In 2000 the US National Intelligence Council (NIC) published *The Global Infectious Disease Threat and Its Implications for the United States*, an unprecedented evaluation of global health issues by the American national security community. The report considers ERIDs a threat to US and global security because diseases will 'endanger US citizens at home and abroad, threaten US armed forces deployed overseas, and exacerbate social and political instability in key countries and regions in which the United States has significant interests' (US National Intelligence Council, 2000). The NIC report is unprecedented because it expands the definition of national security to include threats from selected infections. Notably, it remains firmly focused at the state level, and on the national security of the US.

The focus on the state in most national security thinking provides a strong contrast to the focus on the individual in medicine, and the community in global health. The reason for addressing ERIDs in the NIC report, and in other recent national security analyses of health issues, is their potentially wider political and economic consequences. While these analyses acknowledge the humanitarian dimensions of disease and ill health, their focus is on impacts large enough to affect the national political and economic interests of other states.

The policy response to ERIDs has involved support for the same measures for identifying and responding to bioterrorism – a strong global disease surveillance and monitoring system, backed by effective domestic public health systems. David Heymann, former Executive Director of Communicable Diseases at WHO, argues that this is actually the central pillar of global health security. He writes, 'strengthened capacity to detect and contain naturally caused outbreaks is the only rational way to defend the world against the threat of a bioterrorist attack' (Heymann, 2003). A number of mechanisms have thus been put into place to improve global responses to naturally occurring and deliberately caused disease outbreaks. The Global Outbreak Alert and Response Network and the revision of the International Health Regulations are two such mechanisms.

HIV/AIDS

In 2000, an unprecedented UN Security Council (UNSC) meeting was held on the impact of HIV/AIDS on peace and security in Africa. This was the first time that the UNSC, a body charged with maintaining international peace and security, addressed a health issue. As President of the UNSC at the time, the US narrowly defined the scope of the meetings to gain the approval from other Council members to address the issue. United States Ambassador Holbrooke argued that it was the cruellest irony to send peacekeepers to stop conflict during which they unintentionally spread HIV. In July 2000 the UNSC passed Resolution 1308 requesting further training of peacekeepers on preventing the spread of HIV/AIDS, and encouraging UN member states to increase HIV prevention, testing and treatment for those deployed on peacekeeping missions.

Resolution 1308 directly resulted in a UN training programme to ensure that all peacekeepers receive information about HIV and the creation of a new UNAIDS Office on AIDS, Security and Humanitarian Response. Perhaps more important than the resolution itself was the discussion of HIV/AIDS at the highest levels of national government and within the security community. By bringing the debate to such a venue, the meetings greatly increased the political profile of HIV/AIDS, aiding the founding of the Global Fund to Fight AIDS, Tuberculosis and Malaria in 2002 and other efforts to fight the disease.

HIV/AIDS as a risk to the military and peacekeeping forces

'AIDS is now the leading cause of death in military and police forces in some African countries, accounting for more than half of in-service mortality.' Nwokoji and Ajuwon (2004)

Following the UNSC meetings, various actors supported or objected to the linking of HIV/AIDS and security. Supporting arguments fell into three related categories. The first, and most direct security concern, is that HIV undermines armed forces. Rates of HIV infection are consistently higher among military personnel than the civilian population. UNAIDS (1998: 3) states that sexually transmitted disease 'rates among armed forces are generally 2 to 5 times higher than in civilian populations; in time of conflict the difference can be 50 times higher or more.' In countries with high rates of HIV, the military and police forces may confront a series of HIV-related problems (Table 11.2). Armed forces may lose highly trained personnel while facing a decreasing pool of healthy recruits. Armed forces may also incur high costs to treat soldiers with HIV, leading the military to seek greater proportions of public expenditure (Elbe, 2003). These factors together will affect the operational efficiency of highly affected militaries. Heinecken (2001a) argues that high rates of HIV in militaries will render them less able to protect national and international interests. The International Crisis Group (2001) suggests government inaction on treating HIV may trigger *coups d'état*, and that the perception that a country's military is weakened by HIV/AIDS may trigger military attack. Elbe (2003) however, cautions that the impact of HIV on armed forces is likely to be complex and there is no evidence to date that HIV has inspired armed conflict.

Table 11.2 HIV prevalence within selected African armed forces and date of estimate

Country	HIV prevalence	Date of estimate
Angola	50%	1999
Botswana	33%	1999
Congo (Brazzaville)	10–25%	1999
Cote d'Ivoire	10–20%	1999
Democratic Republic of the Congo	50%	1999
Eritrea	10%	1999
Lesotho	40%	1999
Malawi	50%	1999
Namibia	16%	1999
Nigeria	10–20%	1999
South Africa	15–20%	2000
Swaziland	48%	1997
Tanzania	15–30%	1999
Zambia	60%	1998
Zimbabwe	55%	1999

Source: Heinecken (2001b); US National Intelligence Council (2000).

Data on HIV/AIDS in the armed forces, and UNSC meetings on HIV/AIDS led to growing fears that peacekeeping operations could be threatened. In addition to the concern that peacekeepers themselves spread HIV, high rates of HIV among the militaries in troop contributing countries may make it more difficult to staff peace-keeping missions because countries are unable to spare personnel. High rates of HIV in the South African and Nigerian militaries, major contributors of peace-keeping troops, may imperil African-led responses to regional crises. Countries may be less willing to contribute to peacekeeping operations if they believe their solders will return from a mission infected with HIV. There are cases of soldiers becoming infected from the peacekeeping operations in Cambodia in 1993 and Sierra Leone in 1997 (Elbe, 2003). A final complication is that countries may object to hosting peacekeepers that come from high prevalence countries. In 2001, Eritrea demanded that no HIV positive troops would be deployed in peacekeeping operations on the border of Ethiopia and Eritrea (Elbe, 2003). By both preventing countries from contributing peacekeepers, and limiting some countries' willingness to accept peacekeepers, the HIV/AIDS pandemic may have a major impact on peacekeeping operations.

HIV and political stability

'We are threatened with extinction. People are dying in chillingly high numbers. It is a crisis of the first magnitude.' Festus Mogae, President of Botswana (Rollnick, 2002)

The third and least researched argument linking HIV/AIDS and security is that the disease potentially threatens the political and economic stability of high-burden countries, and may even cause states to fail. Elbe (2003) writes that state failure is a multifaceted process, involving the failure of the economy, political and social institutions. High rates of HIV can contribute to failures in each of these areas. By increasing government spending to prevent and treat HIV/AIDS, decreasing productivity by affecting those in the most productive years of life, and reducing macroeconomic growth, HIV may severely undermine a state's economy. HIV may stress political stability if large numbers of bureaucrats, police officers, teachers, doctors and other essential workers die of AIDS. Unequal access to treatment, based on social, ethnic or political criteria could place unmanageable pressure on political structures. Finally with an expected 20 million AIDS orphans in sub-Saharan Africa by 2010, HIV/AIDS may undermine the family unit. AIDS orphans may have little educational or economic opportunities, and may turn to crime, become radicalized, or even be recruited as child soldiers.

The repercussions of HIV for state stability would differ by country and region. To date, sub-Saharan Africa has been the most highly affected region, and the pandemic could represent a direct national security threat to countries in the region. However before 9/11, the huge human cost of the disease in sub-Saharan Africa was not sufficient to seriously engage powerful countries. Eberstadt (2002) offers a realist perspective:

'Africa's AIDS catastrophe is a humanitarian disaster of world historic proportions, yet the economic and political reverberations from this crisis have been remarkably muted outside the continent itself. The explanation for this awful dissonance lies in the region's marginal status in global economics and politics ... The states of the region are thus not well positioned to influence events much beyond their own borders under any circumstances, good or ill – and the cruel consequence is that the world pays them little attention.'

What has changed is the security environment in the wake of 11 September 2001. Previously, security threats emanated from strong states, countries with leadership, wealth and weapons. 11 September demonstrated that weak states could threaten powerful states by providing safe harbour to terrorist groups. HIV/AIDS and its potential role in undermining state stability has thus put sub-Saharan Africa and other neglected regions onto the security agenda.

A second argument has focused on the security concerns of the US by arguing that a 'second wave' of HIV/AIDS could destabilize nations outside of sub-Saharan Africa that are critical to American strategic interests and global stability. The nations typically included in this group are India, China, and Russia (see Figure 11.2). These are three of the seven declared nuclear states, and their combined population and economic power is substantial. Instability in any of these countries would have major political, economic and military repercussions. That state instability and failure could be caused by HIV/AIDS, in both sub-Saharan Africa and other regions of strategic importance, is a key argument aimed at convincing realists of the threat of the HIV/AIDS pandemic.

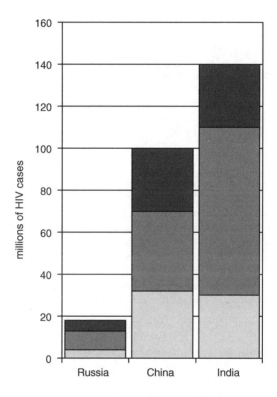

	Mild epidemic	Intermediate epidemic	Severe epidemic
China	32 million	70 million	100 million
India	30 million	110 million	140 million
Russia	4 million	13 million	19 million

Figure 11.2 Projected cumulative new HIV cases, 2000–2025 for Russia, India and China
Source: Eberstadt (2002).

✎ **Activity 11.2**

Think about the arguments used to link the HIV/AIDS pandemic to national security concerns. Choose another major global public health issue of your choice (examples can be found throughout this book). How does the issue meet the three following criteria discussed above?

- pose a severe risk to social well-being by impacting population health status, the health status of a strategic group such as the armed forces, or the economy;
- have an impact across borders and notably in strategically important countries; or
- be an acute threat in a relatively immediate timeframe.

Write a one-page letter to the editor of a health journal arguing why your global health issue is or is not a national security threat.

 Feedback

Some interesting global public health issues you might wish to test are the global obesity epidemic, lack of access by the poor to essential drugs or the health consequences of global environmental change (GEC). The first two, for example, satisfy the first two criteria but not the third. Depending on the nature of the GEC, it may satisfy all three criteria.

Risks and benefits of linking health and security

The recent characterization of global health issues as security threats has resulted in greater political attention and funding to address bioterrorism and selected infectious diseases. This attention has allowed considerable scaling up of global health activities. The coming together of the health and security communities seems mutually favourable, and has been embraced by many leaders in global health. However the long-term implications of global health's move into the areas of security and high politics are unclear.

Viewing HIV/AIDS and other health issues through the lens of security has been criticized by observers within both camps. Objections within the security community concern the overly broad definition of security. A common refrain is that 'if everything is a security issue, then nothing is.' Moreover, it is argued that the link between health and security is speculative, too indirect, and inappropriately concerned with non-military threats.

The global health and development aid communities have also begun to question the securitization of health. Some worry about making global health activities subservient to narrow national interests, and into a tool to pursue foreign policy. For example, there are concerns that funding for public health development could be focused on countries supportive of the so-called 'War on Terror' and other security policy initiatives, instead of based on humanitarian need.

Despite these criticisms, the linkages between global health and national security policy continue to deepen. This will require those in global health to engage more effectively with the security policy community to ensure a strong role for global health in world affairs.

Activity 11.3

Consider once again the global public health issue selected in Activity 11.2. Are there advantages or disadvantages to the public health community of addressing this issue as a threat to national security? What positive or negative effects do you think the security community could experience in incorporating selected health problems into its agenda?

Feedback

In considering the above, you will need to think about what different goals and perspectives the public health and security communities might have, as well as their different degrees of influence over the political agenda. The public health community might benefit from the raising of selected health issues higher on the public policy agenda. However, this might be at the expense of skewing the agenda and thus neglecting other, equally pressing, public health needs. The security community could benefit from dealing in a timely and appropriate manner with a real threat to a population's well-being. However, it may also be seen as risking the opening up of the security agenda too broadly.

Summary

You have learnt about the recent linking of health and security by various scholarly and policy communities which has arisen amid recognition of the global nature of certain health issues, notably infectious diseases and bioterrorism. This should have encouraged you to be more critical in reflecting on the relevance and appropriateness of placing health and security in closer proximity.

References

Commission on Human Security (2003) *Human Security Now*. New York: 159.

Daulaire N (2003) 'Global Health in the Post 9–11 World.' *Harvard Health Policy Review*, 4(1).

Eberstadt N (2002) 'The Future of AIDS.' *Foreign Affairs*, 81(6): 22–45.

Elbe S (2003) *Strategic implications of HIV/AIDS*. Oxford: Oxford University Press.

Heinecken L (2001a) 'HIV/AIDS, the military and the impact on national and international security.' *Society in Transition*, 32(1): 120–7.

Heinecken L (2001b) 'Living in Terror: The Looming Security Threat to Southern Africa.' *African Security Review*, 10(4).

Henderson DA (1998) 'Bioterrorism as a public health threat.' *Emerging Infectious Diseases*, 4(3): 488–92.

Heymann DL (2003) 'The Evolving Infectious Disease Threat: Implications for National and Global Security.' *Journal of Human Development*, 4(2): 191–207.

International Crisis Group (2001) *HIV/AIDS as a Security Issue*. International Crisis Group: 28.

Lippmann W (1943) *US foreign policy: shield of the republic*. Boston: Little, Brown & Company.

Nwokoji UA and Ajuwon AJ (2004) 'Knowledge of AIDS and HIV risk-related sexual behavior among Nigerian naval personnel.' *BMC Public Health*, 4(1): 24.

Poste G (2002) 'Facing reality in preparing for biological warfare: a conversation with George Poste. Interview by Jeff Goldsmith.' *Health Aff (Millwood) Suppl Web Exclusives*: W219–28.

Rollnick R (2002) 'Botswana's high-stakes assault on AIDS.' *Africa Recovery*, 16(2–3): 4–8.

US National Intelligence Council (2000) 'National intelligence estimate: the global infectious disease threat and its implications for the United States.' *Environ Change Secur Proj Rep*, 6: 33–65.

Ullman RH (1983) 'Redefining security.' *International Security*, 8(1): 129–53.

United Nations Development Programme (1994) *Human Development Report 1994, New Dimensions of Human Security* Oxford: Oxford University Press.

Wolfers A (1952) ' "National security" as an ambiguous symbol.' *Political Science Quarterly*, 67(4): 481–502.

Health, globalization and governance: an introduction to public health's 'new world order'

Overview

In this chapter you will focus on the importance of governance to the pursuit of public health in the era of globalization. The chapter defines governance and provides a historical overview of how governance activities for public health have changed. You will learn that the most recent change, which occurred in response to the latest stage of globalization, has taken public health governance in new directions, the implications of which are still unfolding.

Learning objectives

After working through this chapter, you will be able to:

- define governance and distinguish it from government
- identify different levels of governance important for public health
- describe the characteristics of different frameworks for public health governance that have developed historically
- understand how and why public health governance shifted from one framework to the next in the face of new health concepts and challenges
- understand how the latest framework for public health governance operates through examination of a specific infectious disease outbreak
- relate governance frameworks to other issues and problems addressed in this book
- consider problems that confront the new governance context for public health.

Key terms

Anarchy The condition under which sovereign states interact with each other without recognizing any common, superior authority over their individual and collection actions.

Classical regime The international governance framework that developed in the first century of international health diplomacy.

Global governance Governance among states (including intergovernmental organizations) and non-state actors (e.g. non-governmental organizations and multinational corporations).

Global health governance Governance efforts among states and non-state actors for purposes of protecting and promoting human health.

Global public goods for health Products or services connected to promoting or protecting health that exhibit a significant degree of non-rivalry and non-excludability in consumption across national boundaries and traditional regional groupings.

Governance The process of governing, or of controlling, managing or regulating the affairs of some entity.

Government The institutions and procedures for making and enforcing rules and other collective decisions. A narrower concept than the state, which includes the judiciary, military and religious bodies.

Horizontal governance Governance by means of cooperation between sovereign states.

Human right to health The right of individuals to the highest attainable standard of health.

International governance The process of governing the relations between states that involves only the states as legitimate actors.

International law The body of rules that regulates the interactions of states and, in certain situations, the relationships between individuals and the state.

National governance Governance that takes place within a single sovereign state.

Neo-Westphalian governance The return of Westphalian governance characteristics in health policy in the 1990s and early 2000s.

Post-Westphalian governance The governance framework that developed in international health policy after the Second World War under the influence of the World Health Organization.

Public-private partnerships Formal or informal joint endeavours involving state and non-state actors typically focused on a particular health policy issue or problem.

Sovereignty Supreme, exclusive power over the territory and people of a state.

Vertical governance Governance that involves state and non-state actors above and below the sovereign state.

Westphalian governance The framework for governing the relations among sovereign states that developed from the tenets of the Peace of Westphalia (1648).

 Activity 12.1

Public health authorities in the (fictional) country of Sednapolis have identified a cluster of highly unusual illnesses. Preliminary investigations suggest the cause of the illnesses might be infectious and resistant to broad-spectrum antibiotics. The region in which the outbreak has occurred is the economic heart of the country and accounts for most of the country's export and import trade, as well as employing large numbers of immigrant workers. You work for the public health authority in Sednapolis and are asked to respond to this outbreak. Suggest what actors, norms and processes you think Sednapolis should utilize or incorporate in its response. For actors, list individuals, entities or organizations you think need to be involved. For norms, list what rules, principles and guidelines (formal or informal) are relevant to organizing the response. For processes, list mechanisms and activities that might be needed to mount a response.

 Feedback

Thinking about what actors, norms and processes the outbreak in Sednapolis would implicate should introduce you to the *diversity, multiplicity* and *complexity* that characterizes health governance in the era of globalization. You should have included public and private sector actors, different normative motivations for action against the outbreak, and multiple channels through which the actors could respond to the outbreak. If you tended to include only actors within one state (e.g. different ministries of the Sednapolis government), try to think beyond the sovereign state and beyond public actors. Review whether you identified norms that might conflict with each other and cause tension in policy addressing the outbreak. Did the processes that you identified rely strictly on public governmental bodies or did they include a major role for private actors, such as scientists and employers?

Governance: responding to health risks and opportunities

Activity 12.1 asked you to respond to the outbreak of a mysterious illness in a region of a country characterized by cross-border trade and human mobility. Organizing such responses is the objective of public health governance. Generally, *governance* is defined as *the process of governing, or of controlling, managing or regulating the affairs of some entity*. The entity in question could be a country, corporation, hospital or university. *Public health governance* means, thus, *the process of controlling, managing or regulating public and private activities in order to protect and promote population health*.

Assessment of the impacts of globalization on health – both positive and negative – includes considering whether societies individually and collectively are controlling, managing and regulating public and private activities that affect health effectively. Most controversies concerning the relationship between health and the World Trade Organization (WTO) are, in fact, disagreements about how to govern the health-trade linkage.

The controversies surrounding the WTO illustrate how *public health governance* has risen in importance in national and international politics in the last decade. Health as a governance issue has gone from neglect to concern, which signals an important change in the relationship between health and globalization.

Governance involves two activities: procedural and substantive. Procedural aspects of governance focus on actors and how actors interact. In Activity 12.1, you identified actors and processes implicated by the outbreak in Sednapolis – the procedural aspects for governance. You may have listed states and pharmaceutical companies as relevant actors and diplomacy with neighbouring countries and multilateral cooperation through the World Health Organization (WHO) as appropriate mechanisms.

Substantive aspects of governance concern objectives. When you identified norms in Activity 12.1, you were thinking about what goals the effort should seek to achieve. Obviously, controlling the outbreak would be a governance objective. But, Sednapolis may want to control the outbreak for different reasons – to protect the country's economy, to fulfil the human right to health, or to avoid the embarrassment of, and challenges against, the country's leadership.

Governance and government

In Activity 12.1, you probably identified government actors to involve in the outbreak response. Many people equate governance with government, which is a mistake, especially concerning governance in a globalized world. Government is an aspect of governance, but the two are not identical.

Review your response to Activity 12.1, focusing on actors you identified that cannot be considered governments or government agencies – actors such as international organizations (e.g. WHO, WTO), pharmaceutical companies or non-governmental organizations (NGOs). In addition, locate processes that involve interactions between Sednapolis and governments of other countries (e.g. diplomacy). You should understand that no single government exists that can control, manage or regulate Sednapolis's outbreak.

To clarify the point, recall that Sednapolis' outbreak is globalized – the economic links between the region affected and the rest of the world, the labour migration into Sednapolis, and the prospect of an infectious, resistant microbe spreading in this climate of mobile products and people. If you equated governance with government, then, by definition, you could not have governance of Sednapolis's outbreak because no world government exists to address the threat.

States interact in a condition of *anarchy*. Anarchy does not mean chaos; rather, in analysis of international relations, it means that states recognize no common, superior authority. Although no world government exists, relations among states interacting in a condition of anarchy can be organized and structured, and thus governed.

Levels of governance

Understanding the distinction between governance and government allows you to identify levels of governance: *national governance, international governance* and *global governance*. Table 12.1 provides definitions and public health examples of each governance level.

International governance is distinct from national governance because it involves interactions between and among states rather than just activities confined to one country. Global governance differs from international governance because the process involves non-state actors as well as states and intergovernmental organizations. To solidify these analytical distinctions, revisit your response to Activity 12.1

Table 12.1 Levels of governance

Governance level	Definition	Public health example
National governance	Governance within a single state	National sanitary reform efforts by European states in the nineteenth century
International governance	Governance among sovereign states (which includes intergovernmental organizations)	International sanitary treaties (latter half of the nineteenth and first half of the twentieth centuries) and WHO's International Health Regulations
Global governance	Governance among states (including intergovernmental organizations) and non-state actors (e.g. NGOs and multinational corporations)	Global Fund to Fight AIDS, Tuberculosis, and Malaria

Table 12.2 Governance levels and Sednapolis outbreak

Governance level	Definition	Examples from Activity 12.1
National governance	Governance within a single state	
International governance	Governance among sovereign states (which includes intergovernmental organizations)	
Global governance	Governance among states (including intergovernmental organizations) and non-state actors (e.g. NGOs and multinational corporations)	

and divide the governance response you contemplated into these governance levels (use Table 12.2).

In all likelihood, you identified examples from each governance level. Although each level is distinct, each is interdependent. To paraphrase the English philosopher John Donne (1572–1631), no level of governance is an island, especially in a world characterized by globalization.

Westphalian governance and public health's emergence as an international issue

The interdependence that prevails today has not always characterized public health governance in international relations. This section provides an overview of the development of public health governance in international relations. The analysis focuses on the emergence of two frameworks – the *Westphalian* and *post-Westphalian governance frameworks*.

'As an event in the history of international relations the Treaty of Westphalia symbolically indicated a sea-change in international organization – the transition to a system of sovereign states, as sovereigns subject to no higher or competing authority and conveniently determining the number and character of their legal relations with each other.' (Harding and Lim, 1999)

Governance efforts to deal with threats to population health, particularly infectious diseases, are as old as the origins of the modern territorial state, as illustrated by the emergence of quarantine in fourteenth-century Italian city-states. For centuries, such efforts were organized under a framework that derives from the Peace of Westphalia of 1648, which ended the Thirty Years War in Europe. The Peace of Westphalia was seminal for international relations because it established governance principles that have dominated international relations for three centuries and that provided the context into which public health emerged as a diplomatic issue in the mid-nineteenth century.

In Westphalian governance, the only legitimate actors are states. Relations between states are regulated according to three principles:

- *the principle of sovereignty* – a state rules supreme over its territory and people;
- *the principle of non-intervention* – no state should interfere in the domestic affairs of other states;
- *the principle of consent-based international law* – the relations among sovereign states can only be regulated through rules to which the states have given their consent to be bound.

These principles operated through processes – diplomacy, trade and war – dominated by the great powers. Westphalian governance recognized the clout of the great powers and accorded them special prerogatives, such as maintaining the balance of power and managing order in the international system.

Westphalian principles established *horizontal governance* between states. States are the only legitimate actors; and, because the principles of sovereignty and non-intervention render what happens inside a state's territory off-limits, the coverage of Westphalian governance only concerns the regulation of state interaction in the anarchical space between borders (Figure 12.1).

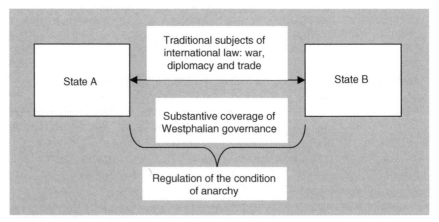

Figure 12.1 Westphalian, horizontal governance
Source: Fidler, 2004.

Public health as a governance issue emerged into the Westphalian system. The Westphalian framework created space for national governance on public health that was off-limits in terms of diplomacy and international law. In terms of relations between states, public health arose as a diplomatic issue in the mid-nineteenth century through the cross-border movement of infectious diseases (e.g. cholera, which hit European countries in a wave of epidemics in the nineteenth century). States responded to the importation of infectious diseases with national governance efforts to reform sanitary systems. But states also responded by implementing quarantine measures on foreign commerce in an attempt to keep infectious diseases out of their territories. In the Westphalian framework, infectious diseases represented exogenous threats to the state to be guarded against (see Figure 12.2).

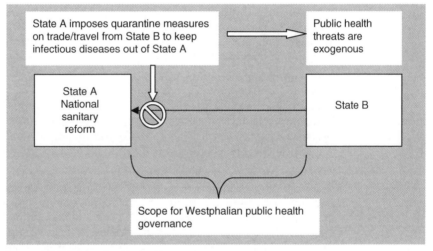

Figure 12.2 National public health governance

In this framework, State A's efforts to keep infectious diseases out of its territory have, however, a reciprocal effect. State B likewise subjects State A's trade and travel to quarantine. State A and State B dislike the burdens the other country's quarantine measures impose on its trade and commerce. States A and B have contradictory objectives in this system of uncoordinated national governance responses: they want to keep foreign germs out, but they want to regulate the ability of other states to keep foreign germs out of their jurisdictions. The only way to reconcile these objectives was to engage in international cooperation, which began to happen in the mid-nineteenth century, starting with the first International Sanitary Conference in 1851.

Through international sanitary conferences and treaties, stretching from the mid-nineteenth century to the Second World War, states abandoned trying to address infectious diseases through uncoordinated national governance. The emergence of international governance reflected: (1) states' realization that their vulnerability to disease importation could not be mitigated effectively without the cooperation of other countries; and (2) the national governance-only approach was increasing economic burdens on international commerce as national efforts to deal with globalizing health risks escalated.

The classical regime

International governance for public health took a particular form, shaped by the over-arching Westphalian framework – *the classical regime*, which represents the most important governance mechanism created during this period. The classical regime appears in the old international sanitary treaties adopted prior to the Second World War and in the International Health Regulations (IHR), originally promulgated by WHO in 1951 and which are still in force today.

The classical regime's purpose was to provide maximum security against the international spread of disease with minimum interference with international trade and travel. Maximum security against international disease spread was to be achieved through binding obligations on states to notify each other directly, or through relevant international health organizations, of the outbreak of specific diseases.

Minimum interference with trade and travel was to be achieved by identifying maximum restrictions that a state could apply against the trade and travel of a state experiencing problems with specified diseases. These maximum measures were based on public health and scientific information concerning the most effective way to prevent disease importation and spread and were designed to enable robust public health action with the least possible interference with world commerce.

Figure 12.3 illustrates the logic of the classical regime: State A agrees to notify State B about a disease outbreak in its territory as long as State B agrees not to impose excessive and irrational measures on State A's trade and commerce. Similarly, State B agrees to so limit its response only if State A alerts it to outbreaks that might spread to State B. Note also that the classical regime is classically Westphalian: (1) the only actors are states; (2) the classical regime contained no provisions about, and showed no interest in, public health conditions inside states; and (3) the classical regime is laid down in consent-based rules of international law.

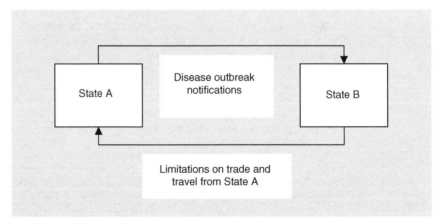

Figure 12.3 The classical regime

The classical regime was also Westphalian in its political dynamics. The diseases subject to the rules of the classical regime were diseases of concern to the great powers because these powers felt vulnerable to the importation of these exogenous disease threats from less-developed countries. Howard-Jones (1950) described European fear of, and diplomatic action against, the importation of 'Asiatic diseases' such as cholera and plague as having flowed 'not from a wish for the general betterment of the health of the world, but the desire to protect certain favoured (especially European) nations from contamination by the less-favoured (especially Eastern) fellows'.

More importantly, what drove the classical regime was the great powers' desire to reduce the burden that foreign quarantine measures imposed on their export trade. Howard-Jones (1975), again: '... the first faltering steps towards international health cooperation followed trade'.

The preamble of the International Sanitary Convention of 1903 (1903 ISC) lists the states present at the International Sanitary Conference that adopted the Convention, and provides that these states have 'deemed it expedient to establish in a single arrangement the measures calculated to safeguard the public health against the invasion and propagation of plague and cholera'. In addition, the 1903 ISC authorized France to submit proposals concerning the establishing of an international health bureau (Article 181), the mandate of which 'shall be to gather information on the development of infectious diseases' (Annex III). The International Office of Public Health was established in 1907, the first world-wide health intergovernmental health organization.

In 1948, the World Health Organization was established through its Constitution. The WHO Constitution's preamble states:

'The States Parties to this Constitution declare ... that the following principles are basic to the happiness, harmonious relations and security of all peoples:

Health is a state of complete physical, mental and social well-being and not merely the absence of disease or infirmity.

The enjoyment of the highest attainable standard of health is one of the fundamental rights of every human being without distinction of race, religion, political belief, economic or social condition.

The health of all peoples is fundamental to the attainment of peace and security and is dependent upon the fullest co-operation of individuals and States.

The achievement of any State in the promotion and protection of health is of value to all.

Unequal development in different countries in the promotion of health and control of disease, especially communicable disease, is a common danger.

Health development of the child is of basic importance; the ability to live harmoniously in a changing total environment is essential to such development.

The extension to all peoples of the benefits of medical, psychological and related knowledge is essential to the fullest attainment of health.

Informed opinion and active co-operation on the part of the public are of the utmost importance in the improvement of the health of the people.

Governments have a responsibility for the health of their peoples which can be fulfilled only by the provision of adequate health and social measures.'

 Activity 12.2

Compare the principles in the WHO preamble with the conception for an international health bureau found in the 1903 ISC. Identify differences and similarities between the 1903 ISC and the WHO Constitution's preamble, in terms of actors, norms and processes.

 Feedback

Conceptions of governance for health internationally radically changed between the 1903 ISC and the preamble of the WHO Constitution. The 1903 ISC and the 1948 WHO Constitution are seminal treaties in the history of health policy and governance, and they reflect significantly different world views of what health means and how governance within and among states needs to be organized to protect and promote health and other interests.

Post-Westphalian public health governance

A major shift from the Westphalian framework toward a new vision of public health in international affairs appears in the WHO Constitution's preamble. Comparing the WHO Constitution's preamble with provisions in the International Sanitary Convention of 1903 introduces a way of thinking about public health governance that rejects Westphalian tenets and bears no resemblance to the classical regime.

Compare the WHO Constitution's preamble with the principles of Westphalian governance on which the classical regime was built. The WHO Constitution's preamble moves governance in a new direction. First, the preamble conceives of public health governance in terms that go beyond the sovereign state and its interests and thus rejects the Westphalian state-centric outlook.

The proclamation that 'the enjoyment of the highest attainable standard of health is one of the fundamental rights of every human being' places individuals, not states, at the centre of governance. The principle that 'the health of all peoples is fundamental to the attainment of peace and security' indicates that this new vision shifts the focus from the state to peoples.

Second, the WHO Constitution's preamble demonstrates concern with public health inside states, which breaks with the Westphalian framework's lack of attention on such conditions. The declaration that health is a human right opens national governance to scrutiny. This perspective clashes with the principle of non-interference in the domestic affairs of states. The pronouncement that 'governments have a responsibility for the health of their peoples which can be fulfilled only by the provision of adequate health measures' likewise focuses on how states organize their health policies internally.

Third, the WHO Constitution's preamble draws inspiration not from consent-based international law but from natural law concepts of individual rights, human solidarity and universal justice. The *human right to health* cannot be found in Westphalian international law. Similarly, the preamble's perspective on health and human solidarity is not Westphalian: 'Unequal development in different countries in the promotion of health and control of disease, especially communicable disease, is a common danger.'

The WHO Constitution's preamble contains a *post-Westphalian* vision for public health governance. This concept promotes a *vertical governance strategy* different from the Westphalian *horizontal governance* approach. The post-Westphalian framework attempts a vertical re-allocation of governance power away from the state and toward governance authority for WHO and governance power for non-state actors – citizens – as holders of the right to health. Sovereignty is penetrated from above and below in order to mitigate public health threats as close to their source as possible and to ensure individuals the highest attainable standard of health.

Post-Westphalian public health governance in action

During the Cold War, the post-Westphalian content of the WHO Constitution's preamble informed WHO policy. The preamble represents more than rhetoric in terms of how WHO organized its activities. The move away from Westphalian governance can be detected in four themes in WHO's work in the Cold War period:

- WHO became more interested in addressing infectious diseases at their local sources through eradication campaigns (e.g. smallpox) than in trying to govern cross-border microbial traffic.
- WHO focused on health problems within developing countries, rather than protecting the great powers' trading interests.
- WHO launched 'Health for All' in the late 1970s in order to build a framework for the realization of the right to health through universal access to primary health care. Health for All is light years from the Westphalian perception of public health threats as exogenous problems for the health and trade of the great powers.
- WHO linked Health for All to demands by the developing world in the 1970s for a 'New International Economic Order'.

Twenty years' crisis: public health governance in the 1980s and 1990s

The zenith of the post-Westphalian governance approach launched by the WHO Constitution occurred in the late 1970s, when the WHO celebrated the global eradication of smallpox and the launch of the Health for All campaign. Over the course of the next 20 years, dramatic public health and political developments exposed the limitations of post-Westphalian governance, forcing those interested in advancing global health to search for new governance strategies.

Such dramatic developments included the HIV/AIDS pandemic; the decline in WHO's effectiveness and credibility; the collapse of the New International Economic Order (with which Health for All had been affiliated); the rise of economic globalization in the post-Cold War triumph of liberal and neo-liberal economic models; the world crisis in emerging and re-emerging infectious diseases; the global pandemic of tobacco-related diseases; and the emergence of the World Bank, the International Monetary Fund (IMF), and the WTO. These three institutions have tremendous influence on public health and health care policies in developing countries. As one World Bank official put it, 'The World Bank is the new 800-pound gorilla in world health care' (Abbassi, 1999).

The impact of these developments suggested that neither the traditional Westphalian nor post-Westphalian frameworks provided an appropriate foundation for public health governance in the globalized world. The HIV/AIDS pandemic and the crisis in emerging and re-emerging infectious diseases revealed how irrelevant the classical regime, in the form of WHO's International Health Regulations (IHR), had become. Similarly, the Health for All approach, with its emphasis on the human right to health, human solidarity and universal justice, lost credibility as a platform from which to mount a governance counter-attack against the threats mounting against public health.

The emergence of neo-Westphalianism and a new form of post-Westphalianism

In the 1990s and early 2000s, new thinking emerged within the Westphalian and post-Westphalian frameworks. The Westphalian approach was given new life through a neo-Westphalian outlook tied to the emerging vulnerability of the great powers to the resurgence of infectious diseases and the threat of bioterrorism. A new kind of post-Westphalian approach also appeared, which fostered development of *global health governance* (GHG) to produce *global public goods for health* (GPGH) (Figure 12.4).

Neo-Westphalianism

The Westphalian perspective experienced a renaissance in the 1990s and early 2000s because the great powers, especially the US, became re-engaged with public health policy. During the Cold War, the great powers disengaged from international governance for public health because they had largely managed to improve their national public health sufficiently to believe, mistakenly, that they had conquered infectious diseases. International governance for public health became a 'mere humanitarian' matter unconnected with the strategic self-interests of the great powers.

Three developments changed the political context sufficiently to get the great powers concerned again about public health governance nationally and internationally:

- The great powers began to feel vulnerable to exogenous infectious disease threats. The growing interest in the US in emerging and re-emerging infectious

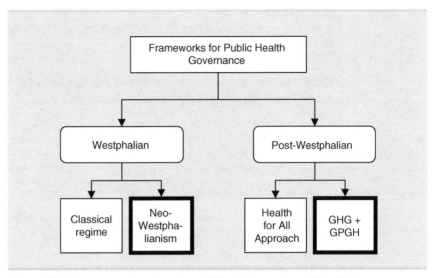

Figure 12.4 Emergence of new branches of Westphalian and post-Westphalian governance

diseases indicated that germs once again had the attention of the great powers in old and new ways. The old way involved the threat of disease importation. The new way concerned worries that infectious diseases in other states, especially HIV/AIDS, could contribute to instability and state failure in strategic countries, such as China, India and Russia.

- The threat of bioterrorism emerged as a new feature that ignited neo-Westphalian interest in public health governance, especially at home. The US and other countries have spent billions of dollars reinforcing and rebuilding their national public health systems in order to prepare effective defences against, and response capabilities for, biological attack – from a few hundred million dollars in 2001 to over 5,000 million dollars in 2004 (US Dept HHS, 2004).
- An older Westphalian feature re-appeared with a new twist. Neo-Westphalianism is partly driven by concerns that the national public health measures of other countries are adversely affecting the trade interests of the great powers. In the Westphalian era, the measures in question involved quarantine. In the neo-Westphalian world, the measures are compulsory licensing and parallel importing of patented pharmaceutical products, which threaten the great powers' efforts to advance a global regime of intellectual property protection for patented drugs and medicines. The controversies concerning the WTO's Agreement on the Trade-Related Aspects of Intellectual Property Rights (TRIPS) illustrate how the Westphalian public health-trade link has emerged in a new guise.

The emergence of a neo-Westphalian perspective can be seen in developments of US policy that have given public health a much higher governance profile than at any other time in the history of the US. The importance of public health to US policy can be seen in many governance areas, including national security, homeland security, foreign policy, trade policy and humanitarian aid. These developments in US foreign policy demonstrate that global health issues are becoming pertinent to the governance considerations of all states, no matter where they sit in the hierarchy of political power.

Global health governance and global public goods for health: a new form of post-Westphalian governance

As neo-Westphalianism was emerging, a new form of post-Westphalian governance developed. The new post-Westphalianism involves a new process – global health governance (GHG) – that seeks to achieve new substantive objectives – global public goods for health (GPGH). This new post-Westphalian strategy differs from the approach outlined in the WHO Constitution's preamble and pursued by WHO during the Cold War.

In terms of the new process of GHG, the strategy involves attempts to integrate non-state actors into public health governance, such as:

- Public-private partnerships for health (e.g. Global Fund to Fight AIDS, Tuberculosis and Malaria).
- Permitting WHO to use non-governmental sources of information for global epidemiological surveillance of infectious diseases (e.g. WHO's Global Outbreak Alert and Response Network), a practice not permitted under the classical regime embodied in the IHR.
- Activating, energizing and involving non-state actors in crafting and implementing new governance regimes, as happened with WHO's Framework Convention on Tobacco Control and proposed with WHO's proposed revision of the IHR.

In traditional post-Westphalianism, non-state actors, predominantly individuals, affected governance because they had a right to claim resources from state actors under the human right to health. In the new post-Westphalianism, non-state actors are not primarily rights-based claimants but are co-producers of goods and services that benefit public health governance at every level. The new post-Westphalianism does not reject the rights-based strategy of Health for All, but neither does it require the rights-based approach to function.

The new post-Westphalian approach operates by focusing GHG mechanisms on the production of GPGH, which are defined as *products or services connected to promoting or protecting health that exhibit a significant degree of non-rivalry and non-excludability in consumption across national boundaries and traditional regional groupings*. GPGH range from global epidemiological surveillance information to new antimicrobials and vaccines.

GHG production is post-Westphalian because it satisfies all the criteria for a post-Westphalian governance approach:

- GPGH production involves state and non-state actors and thus rejects state-centric governance.
- Consumers of GPGH are governmental and non-governmental actors, which again constitutes a rejection of state-centrism.
- GPGH production and consumption often involve efforts that affect public health within countries, which ignores the Westphalian emphasis on sovereignty and non-intervention.

- GPGH production does not depend on the creation of consent-based rules of international law, as illustrated the Global Fund to Fight AIDS, Tuberculosis and Malaria – a Swiss, non-profit organization not based on treaty law or customary international law.
- GPGH production creates goods and services that benefit more than one country and narrowly defined national interests.

SARS as a breakthrough for the new post-Westphalian framework

The management of the outbreak of Severe Acute Respiratory Syndrome (SARS) in 2003 represented a seminal moment for the new post-Westphalian governance framework because this outbreak was controlled through the production of GPGH by GHG.

In terms of GHG, the new post-Westphalian framework appeared during the SARS outbreak in:

- WHO access to, and use of, non-governmental sources of surveillance information, which proved powerful in dealing with China and in creating incentives for other affected states to report SARS cases to WHO and not attempt to cover up their outbreaks.
- WHO leadership in building coalitions of state and non-state actors in tackling SARS-related public health, scientific, clinical treatment and technological challenges.
- WHO issuance of travel alerts and advisories directly to non-state actors – travellers – without consulting the states affected by such measures.

WHO's actions during SARS reflected a radically new governance context for the sovereign state. WHO's access to non-governmental information and its ability to issue travel alerts and advisories squeezes the state's sovereignty concerning how it handles outbreaks of infectious diseases (Figure 12.5). The GHG pincer that unfolded in SARS illustrates how significantly the context in which states exercise sovereignty with respect to infectious diseases has changed in ways that Westphalian concepts cannot explain.

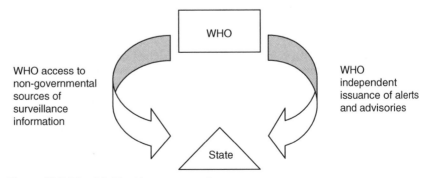

Figure 12.5 The global health governance pincer

Source: Fidler, 2004.

In terms of GPGH, the SARS outbreak also represented a breakthrough moment for the new post-Westphalian governance framework because the outbreak's management illustrated the power of producing GPGH in the context of a public health crisis. WHO led global efforts to produce surveillance data on SARS, design clinical treatment guidelines for SARS patients, conduct research on the causative agent of SARS, and develop diagnostics, therapies and vaccines.

GPGH production in these contexts created a *global health governance platform* to support national governance. As states confronted the GHG pincer, GHG mechanisms built information, scientific, clinical and technological resources to assist state responses to the threat. This post-Westphalian approach creates a governance context in which the political incentives to cooperate, collaborate and coordinate are strong. In this new climate, national, international and global governance integrate in a common effort against a public health threat.

 Activity 12.3

Although the new post-Westphalian framework produced results in the SARS outbreak, this approach may confront difficulties in the future. Identify one public health problem of global concern in the communicable and in the non-communicable disease areas. For each problem, analyse whether GPGH production through GHG has the potential to reduce the threats to public health you identified. Write down whether you think the problems would be better addressed by the Westphalian/ neo-Westphalian frameworks or by the Health for All approach.

 Feedback

You may have struggled to apply the GHG and GPGH concepts to health problems other than SARS. You may have identified ways in which GHG and GPGH could be useful with respect to the disease problems you selected, but you may have also noted that the utility is, at present, more theoretical than real because the needed mechanisms and financial resources have not yet materialized. Governance of the SARS may have been effective, but it may also not be representative of the governance reality that applies to many health problems around the world. Recognizing these gaps in the emerging system is important for stimulating further governance action and innovation.

Coming to terms with public health's 'new world order'

Activity 12.3 encouraged you to think about obstacles that might confront the new post-Westphalian governance framework that emerged in the 1990s and early 2000s, and which had a breakthrough moment in the SARS outbreak. Previous governance innovations (e.g. the move to international governance in the nineteenth century; the development of the classical regime; and the Health for All approach) eventually lost steam, encouraging further experimentation with governance. Does the new post-Westphalianism face the same fate?

You may have identified communicable and non-communicable disease problems for which the approach used against SARS offers less in terms of governance prospects. Is, for example, the strategy used against SARS helpful in addressing the HIV/AIDS epidemic? Similar questions can be asked of non-communicable diseases affecting populations around the world – tobacco-related diseases, exposure to carcinogenic pollutants moving across boundaries, and obesity-related diseases.

Your effort to identify problems that confront the new post-Westphalian public health governance strategy may have been fertile because many problems exist. The existence of problems does not, however, fatally undermine the transition public health governance has experienced in the last decade. In battling SARS, a leading WHO official described this transition as the emergence of a 'new way of working.' Another WHO official likened what happened in SARS to the crossing of a global health Rubicon, after which there was no possibility of returning to the ways of the past. Public health has entered a new world order; but its future yet remains largely undetermined and waiting to be made.

References

Abbassi K (1999) 'Changing Sides'. *British Medical Journal*; 318: 865–9.

Fidler DP (2004) *SARS, Governance, and the Globalization of Disease*. Basingstoke: Palgrave Macmillan.

Harding C and Lim CL (1999) 'The Significance of Westphalia: An Archaeology of the International Legal Order'. In *Renegotiating Westphalia: Essays and Commentary on the European and Conceptual Foundations of Modern International Law* (Harding C and Lim CL, eds). The Hague: M. Nijhoff Publishers: 1–23.

Howard-Jones N (1950) 'Origins of International Health Work'. *British Medical Journal* (6 May), 1032–7.

Howard-Jones N (1975) *The Scientific Background of the International Sanitary Conferences 1851–1938*. Geneva: WHO.

US Department of Health and Human Services (2004) *Fact Sheet: Biodefense Preparedness*, 28 April.

13 The commercial sector and global health governance

Overview

In this chapter you will learn about the involvement of the commercial sector in global health governance. The chapter begins by defining the commercial sector and enumerating the range of commercial entities with an interest in global health. It then differentiates between three distinct pathways through which the commercial sector plays a role in global health: establishing private systems of global health governance; influencing public governance; and involvement in co-regulation with the public sector. Examples of each of these approaches are provided and their strengths and limitations are discussed.

Learning objectives

After working through this chapter, you will be able to:

- **provide examples of formal and informal commercial organizations with an interest in global health**
- **explain why it is important to consider the role of the commercial sector in global health governance**
- **differentiate between three approaches to commercial sector involvement in global health governance**
- **list benefits and risks of the involvement of the commercial sector in global health governance.**

Key terms

Code of conduct Voluntary measure undertaken by a firm to impact upon some aspect of its business practice.

Corporate social responsibility Industry supported measures whereby companies attempt to demonstrate responsible behaviour.

Corporation An association of stockholders which is regarded as an artificial person under most national laws. Ownership is marked by ease of transferability and stockholders have limited liability.

Industry Groups of firms closely related by use of similar technology of production or high level of substitutability of products.

Intellectual property Creations of the mind, including inventions, literary and artistic works, and symbols, names, images and designs. It is of two types: industrial (e.g. patents and trademarks) and copyright (e.g. musical).

> **Regulation** The enforcement of norms, standards, rules and principles which govern behaviour.

What is the commercial sector?

This section clarifies what is meant by the commercial sector and introduces a range of commercially oriented organizations that impact on global health governance (GHG) via the pursuit of their interests. A useful starting point is the common distinction between public and private actors. Here public refers to state, governmental and intergovernmental organizations (e.g. the Government of Burundi or the World Health Organization [WHO]), whereas private is a residual category of all remaining organizations and entities. The commercial sector lies clearly within the private category but is qualitatively different from civil society actors, the latter being marked by their voluntary and non-commercial nature.

The private commercial sector is characterized by its market-orientation. It comprises organizations that seek to make profits for their owners (e.g. firms). Profit, or a return on investment, is the central defining feature of the commercial sector. Many firms pursue additional objectives related, for example, to social, environmental or employee concerns; but these are, of necessity, secondary and supportive of the primary objective. In the absence of profit, firms cease to exist.

In thinking about the role of the commercial sector in GHG it is useful to include organizations that are not-for-profit in their legal status, registered for example, with charitable status, but established to support a firm or industry. These may include business federations, such as the International Federation of Pharmaceutical Manufacturers Associations (IFPMA). Similarly, not-for-profit organizations established by companies or wealthy individuals but run at an arm's length from them (e.g. the Soros Foundation) are included here as many foundations have injected both large quantities of resources and the mindset of commerce into the global health sector.

This broad approach to the commercial sector suggests that organizations belonging to any of the following nine categories could influence GHG:

- Multi- and trans-national corporations with an interest or impact on health (e.g. Pfizer);
- Global cartels in the health sector. Cartels are groups that collude to eliminate competition or increase leverage on policy processes. The existence of a global price fixing cartel for vitamins between 1989 and 1999 resulted in convictions in the EU and the US of several leading pharmaceutical firms;
- Business associations, established to promote their members' interests, may have global health sector interests: the International Chamber of Commerce (ICC) develops 'business policy' in precaution, science and risk, and bio-technology with implications for health; the World Economic Forum, representing the world's 1,000 leading companies, hosts a Global Health Initiative that develops and communicates best practice in the area of HIV/AIDS, TB and malaria;

- Associations of privately employed professionals with an interest in global health. This includes organizations of health care providers, such as the International Private Practitioners Association and other professional associations whose practices or interests impact on health;
- Non-profit standardizing associations covering health-related domains and subject to high levels of industry influence. For example, in relation to standards governing tobacco products (e.g. methods for measuring tar and nicotine yield), the International Standards Organization, a non-profit body, relies heavily on CORESTA, a scientific body, that is run by the tobacco industry;
- Non-profit, issue-specific, industry-funded think-tanks, and institutes with interests in global health. For example, documents from the tobacco company Philip Morris reveal that it provided $US880,000 to create the Institute of Regulatory Policy in the US 'as a vehicle [to lobby] for the executive order on risk assessment', aiming to delay the publication of an EPA report on environmental tobacco smoke (quoted in Muggli et al., 2004);
- Non-profit, 'patient groups' established to advance industry interests. The International Alliance of Patients' Organizations is registered as a charitable foundation in the Netherlands and funded by Pharmaceutical Partners for Better Healthcare, a consortium of about 30 major companies. It has over 100 member patient organizations and a stated interest in improving patient voice. Its hidden agenda is likely to support consumer advertising and public/insurance funding of specific treatments;
- Non-profit, industry-established and industry-funded scientific organizations with an interest in health issues. For example, the International Life Sciences Institute supports industry-friendly science and attempts to influence regulation in areas such as diet, tobacco and alcohol; and
- Non-profit, philanthropic organizations that invest resources in global health, influence global priorities and approaches, and leverage additional commercial sector involvement.

When considering the governance of a global health issue, it is important to assess the different kinds of commercial organizations that may have an impact on it, the influence of such organizations on how the issue is governed, and how proposed reforms to governance may affect commercial interests.

 Activity 13.1

Think about how global governance was defined in Chapter 12. Now look back over the above list. Can you spot the sorts of entities that are missing from the list? Here is a clue: global governance is characterized by formal as well as informal institutional arrangements.

 Feedback

The above list includes only formal organizations. A comprehensive list would need to include less formal groups which promote the interests of the commercial sector in global health, for example:

- Loose issue-oriented networks. ARISE (Associates for Research into the Science of Enjoyment) publishes articles promoting the pleasures of 'smoking, alcohol, caffeine and chocolate', and receives funding from companies such as Coca-Cola, Miller Beer and Kraft;
- More integrated private policy and regulatory communities. The Intellectual Property Committee, a group of 12 Chief Executive Officers largely responsible for one of the WTO trade agreements, provides one such example; and
- Forms of a globalizing commercial sector with an interest in GHG can be found on the Internet in the guise of virtual service providers (e.g. World Directory of Holistic Practitioners, virtual communities, and virtual campaigners. Internet sites can also serve as fronts for commercial organizations. For example, it has been claimed that the Bivings Group, a PR firm employed by Monsanto, established a website for a non-existent research organization to launch campaigns against environmentalists and invented 'phantom citizens' who sent thousands of e-mails and petitions to selected list servers and notice boards.

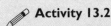 **Activity 13.2**

Select a global health issue with which you are familiar and list the commercial organizations relevant to it. Identify one or two examples for each of the categories listed above. Fill in Table 13.1 by listing the interests of these organizations in the issue, the roles that they play in relation to the issue, and their impact on health.

Table 13.1 Commercial organizations active in a selected global health issue

Type of organization	Name of organizations	Interests in the issue	Roles in the issue	Impact on health
MNC/TNC	1. 2.			
Business associations	1. 2.			
Professional associations	1. 2.			
Standards organizations	1. 2.			
Think tanks	1. 2.			
Patient groups	1. 2.			
Scientific networks	1. 2.			
Philanthropic organizations	1. 2.			
Loose networks	1. 2.			
Tight networks	1. 2.			
Virtual organizations	1. 2.			

Feedback

By now it will be clear that although the commercial sector comprises those organizations established to realize a profit for their owners, consideration of the sector's role in global health also requires recognition of those organizations which may be non-profit but serve corporate ends. By adopting this approach, a vast range of commercially oriented organizations and networks with an interest in global health emerge. The sector is highly differentiated with organizations varying by size, kinds of resources (financial capital, technology, employment and natural resources), level of formalization, geographical scope, compliance with the rule of law, as well as by their interest in GHG.

Globalization and the commercial health sector

Globalization and the private sector are intractably entwined and, for many observers, globalization's economic face is its most familiar – the rise of global brands, companies and products. The growth of transworld spaces has left an indelible mark on the commercial sector by unleashing resources on an unprecedented scale. Indeed, the commercial sector has also been a driving force behind globalization.

Although highly clichéd, the present era is characterized by the emergence of global firms comprising global communications, global markets, brands and products, global production, marketing, advertising and distribution, global consumer culture, global information infrastructure, and the increasing commoditization of various aspects of social and physical existence – including health.

The emergence of a global economy has been characterized by tremendous growth in the number and scale of global firms. In the health sector, these trends apply to pharmaceutical companies, biotechnology companies, medical device firms, health care providers, insurance firms, hospital consortia and so on. In some industries, like pharmaceuticals, recent years have seen both a concentration of ownership and considerable strategic alliance building. Globalization has created a new breed of corporate giant, rivalling the size of some national economies and with a wider reach than some intergovernmental organizations.

Yet globalization also presents a challenge to these global companies: as firms expand their reach, they have an increasing need for rules to govern their transactions on a global basis. Such rules serve to minimize uncertainty and lower transaction costs associated with information gathering, negotiation and enforcement. As early as 1998, the Secretary General of International Chamber of Commerce (ICC) indicated that 'Business believes that the rules of the game for the market economy, previously laid down almost exclusively by national governments, must be applied globally if they are to be effective' (Cattaui, 1998). Where possible, business seeks to establish its own rules – as it has done through the ICC since 1911. Where this is not possible, it seeks to influence public regulation, through, for example, the United Nations.

While firms may look to systems of global governance to improve their fortunes, their involvement in such systems raises questions about how that might impact on public health and public institutions. Before considering these issues, a broader matter concerns the significance of the commercial sector in global health governance.

Activity 13.3

Make a list of reasons why health policy makers should give attention to the role(s) of the commercial sector in global health governance. In framing your response consider the nature of global health problems, the capacity of the state to address them, and the assets of the commercial sector.

Feedback

Your answer might include any of the following considerations.

Health impacts of transborder flows often exceed the regulatory capacity of governments, whether acting alone or collectively through intergovernmental organizations. These include the illicit trade of goods and services (and persons), spread of anti-microbial resistance and pathogens, emerging and re-emerging infectious diseases, environmental pollution, information and communication, and population migration. Since the commercial sector often plays a role in such flows, the need arises to rethink classical state-centric public health approaches to dealing with them. How should the commercial sector be involved in governing these cross-border flows in ways that can contribute to public health goals?

Global health challenges call into question the effectiveness of existing institutions. On the one hand, driven by ideology, resource scarcity and spiralling health care costs, many governments have embarked on ambitious reform programmes, often altering the balance between public and private sectors. These typically involve an enlarged role for commercial organizations in health finance, delivery and governance. On the other hand, public sector institutions involved in global health need to adapt to the changing global environment so as to remain relevant and effective. Many organizations, such as the World Bank and WHO, have strategically engaged in new relationships with the commercial sector in response to this necessity. Such relationships between intergovernmental and commercial organizations, both formal and informal, represent nascent initiatives to govern global health issues.

The commercial sector is simply too large to ignore. Given that the majority of the one hundred largest economies in the world are corporations rather than states, private corporate standards and rules cannot be deemed inconsequential. WHO's biennial budget for 2002–03 was US$2.2 billion. Pfizer, had sales of US$39 billion in 2003, which did not include revenues from its over-the-counter, diagnostic and animal health divisions. Total sales for the top 50 firms was US$466 billion, up from US$296 billion two years earlier. No international organization and few states can deploy resources for research and development on the scale of the pharmaceutical companies.

A fourth argument for a greater role for the commercial sector reflects its potential contribution to GHG. The sector is widely perceived to have a comparative advantage in terms of skills, knowledge, expertise, know-how, and manufacturing, distribution, marketing and branding capability. Perhaps GHG could draw more effectively on private sector expertise to protect and promote health. In product development partnerships, industry provides goods (e.g. compounds, tools and technologies) as well as services such as participation on governing bodies, personnel inputs for project management, technology services, access to proprietary data and information, functional or scientific expertise. Such contributions are increasingly attractive as the commercial sector is generally at the forefront of new technologies. The vast resources of the commercial sector can be, arguably should be, and are increasingly being harnessed to support GHG.

Why a concern with the commercial sector in global health governance?

This book conceptualizes GHG broadly, encompassing diverse formal and informal systems impacting on health – including systems established or dominated by the commercial sector.

Thus companies, given their global reach, may have a comparative advantage over both states and intergovernmental organizations in governing global health issues. This does not mean that the goals of the private and public sectors will necessarily coincide on any given health issue. For example, regarding the marketing of medicines, industry guidelines are more concerned that misleading claims will lead to loss of revenue among more scrupulous companies, whereas WHO guidelines are concerned with patient well-being and cost-efficiency at the population level.

Where private health governance is effective, consistent with public interests, and alleviates the need for public sector governance, it follows that such efforts serve to reduce public sector expenditure. Nonetheless, private governance may be ineffective or have negative consequences for health. This provides a rationale for scrutiny of mechanisms of private sector governance.

The commercial sector and global health governance

Having defined GHG in broad terms and highlighted the diverse engagement of the commercial sector, it is important to distinguish between different kinds of involvement. This chapter advances a conceptual framework that permits categorization of the range and scope of such contributions by identifying three main types of governance involving the private sector: self-regulation; influence on public regulation; and co-regulation.

Self-regulation through private standards

Self-regulation concerns efforts by private companies to establish their own rules and policies for operating within a specific domain. For example, rules governing how to design, categorize, produce and handle goods or services may be adopted by individual companies or industries. These range from the activities of the

International Chamber of Commerce, establishing rules and standards in areas like nomenclature in trade and investment, commercial law, and banking, but also settling disputes through its international court of arbitration, to the ongoing efforts of multiple business associations represented by the Alliance for Global Business to develop standards for e-commerce.

Private market standards may be formally adopted or informally adhered to, and they may be expressed as statements of principles, guidelines, undertakings, codes, declarations or standards. All belong to the category of private- or soft-law, meaning that they are voluntary rather than traceable to public authority. These rules are enforced by market actors and neither monitored nor subject to public verification.

Activity 13.4

1 Self-regulation involves intergovernmental organizations (such as WHO) issuing guidelines which companies must abide by. True/False?
2 Self-regulation is a form of soft-law. True/False?
3 Self-regulation consists solely of instruments which are formally adopted by businesses and industries. True/False?

Feedback

1 False. Self-regulatory guidelines, standards, principles and so on are generally issued by commercial sector organizations.

2 True. Self-regulatory initiatives are not promulgated, monitored or enforced by public authority.

3 False. Self-regulation, like most systems of global governance, comprises both formal or informal mechanisms.

There are two principal types of self-regulation, respectively regulating 'market standards' and 'social standards'. In the case of market standards, products, process and business practice may be subject to governance to support commerce (e.g. to reduce transaction costs or increase confidence in a product). Although such self-regulation may have social impacts, the overriding purpose of market standards is to enable commerce.

There are thousands of examples of industry regulation of market standards, many related to global health – from advertising and public relations codes of conduct to standards on the threads on screws used within medical equipment. For example, private market standards are rapidly developing in electronic health informatics through the Global Information Infrastructure Commission (GIIC). The GIIC is a confederation of Chief Executive Officers (CEOs) of firms that develop and deploy, operate and finance information and communication technology infrastructure. This private commission aims to harmonize global policies through 'business self-regulation'. In 1996, based on the work of the Health Information Infrastructure

Consortium (a group of 110 US-based and multinational institutions), the GIIC published a paper on Healthcare and Telemedicine (GIIC, 1996). The paper covered areas such as:

- administrative information systems, for example, exchange of electronic unified claims forms and other data;
- clinical information systems which access, store and transmit information to enable global access to patient records, claims and clinical protocols;
- personal health information systems (targeting consumers/patients directly); and
- telemedicine.

The paper recommended further development of global rules and harmonization in nomenclature to facilitate the emergence of global markets for health information. The GIIC exemplifies industry efforts to self-regulate market standards.

Private market standards have been established in contexts of weak or non-existent public (or private) regulation of market activity or industry fear of (inter)governmental action. Such standards may have both positive and negative health outcomes (either intended or as an unintended consequence). For example, global rules governing transborder electronic movement of patient records could benefit patients who travel internationally for surgery as 'medical tourists' but could also infringe upon patient confidentiality or increase costs to consumers or insurers through restrictive intellectual property practices.

By contrast, self-regulation through social standards involves business and industry voluntarily adopting and observing specific practices based on public or social concern rather than to improve the functioning of the market. Self-regulatory social standards are usually developed in response to consumer concerns or boycotts, shareholder activism, or the threat of impending public regulation.

Self-regulation of social standards includes corporate social responsibility, voluntary codes and reporting initiatives, and some public-private partnerships. Such standards often address issues that are already subject to (often ineffective) statutory regulation. For example, the International Labour Organization (ILO) has issued standards governing maternity leave and breastfeeding at work; some countries have adopted the standards (e.g. India), others have not (e.g. Kenya), while implementation is often partial.

In practice, it can be difficult to distinguish between self-regulation of market and social standards as some mechanisms pursue both goals. For example, in response to a series of food scandals (e.g. BSE, pesticides, genetically modified foods), EUREPGAP, a consortium of global food companies began developing food safety and hygiene standards. Industry claims that the initiative responds to consumer concerns while others contend that it aims to pre-empt public regulation. Yet the initiative also facilitates global markets, since EUREPGAP's members desire a commonly applied reference standard (www.eurep.org/about.html).

Corporate social responsibility

Corporate social responsibility (CSR) is an umbrella term for diverse self-regulatory measures intended to present firms and industries as operating responsibly in terms of their social impacts. There are now a plethora of social reporting, investment and corporate citizenship initiatives.

The definition of social responsibility remains problematic. Tobacco, arms and alcohol industries might be viewed as incompatible with CSR but not everyone will agree that such companies are intrinsically socially irresponsible. Moreover, for some investors this will be irrelevant as investments will be made on the basis of potential return. For example, returns to investments in a self-named 'Vice Fund' of alcohol, gaming, tobacco and aerospace/defence stocks, are above Standard & Poor's 500 index average. The trade-off between CSR and returns to capital may be difficult to reconcile.

Codes of conduct

Voluntary codes of conduct are the most prominent form of self-regulation of social standards. Companies and industry make public commitments to adhere to a set of standards they themselves set. Codes cover multiple corporate practices that impact on important determinants of health, including workplace and occupational health and safety (e.g. worker exposure to pesticide residues, access to on-site clinics), wages and working hours, minimum working age, forced labour, discrimination, freedom of association, right of collective bargaining, product safety, responsible promotion, advertising and marketing (e.g. over-the-counter medications, breast-milk substitutes), hygiene and food safety, protection of the environment, and human rights.

Codes have proliferated and by the turn of the century most global firms and industry sectors had adopted codes, many of which are global in reach. For example, member companies of the IFPMA are asked to adhere to the Federation's Code of Pharmaceutical Marketing Practice, while major tobacco companies have recently developed International Tobacco Marketing Standards.

 Activity 13.5

Why might a company commit itself to adhering to a voluntary code? Suggest four to five reasons.

 Feedback

While serving social purposes, codes can serve important business functions and ultimately increase profits. Your answer should include some of the following reasons why codes may improve profitability:

- demonstrate responsiveness to societal concerns;
- provide material for public relations;
- differentiate itself from competitors to increase sales;
- respond to concerns of consumers to increase sales;
- respond to concerns of shareholders and encourage greater investment;

- decrease costs. The British mining conglomerate, Anglo American PLC, estimates that 30,000 of its employees in South Africa are infected with HIV. It has voluntarily adopted a code in relation to treatment of 3,000 employees, costs being reportedly offset by sharp decline in mortality and absenteeism due to illness;
- stave off or delay statutory regulation. The tobacco, pharmaceutical and food safety codes mentioned above were advanced to pre-empt more onerous international obligations; and
- provide flexible tools tailored to specific problems instead of blanket regulations covering all contingencies.

Voluntary codes may not only be good for business. Codes can bring new stakeholders into the regulatory process. For example, temporary labourers, often women, have participated in developing workplace codes, having not typically been represented in comparable ILO processes. Second, codes may generate better compliance than public regulation. Experience with many international conventions governing social and economic issues suggests that ratifying governments often fail to implement them, and cannot be held accountable by the international community for such failure. In theory, companies adopt codes to gain market share and comply with them to retain the confidence of their consumers/shareholders. Third, codes are less costly to the public sector than statutory regulation.

There are, however, reasons for scepticism regarding the ability of voluntary codes to adequately govern many global health issues. One review of a large number of codes concludes that codes typically comprise lofty statements of intent, are largely responsive to consumer pressure and highlight issues in consumer-sensitive industries (e.g. apparel) while ignoring many others. Moreover, companies generally lack the means to communicate compliance in reliable and believable ways. Codes have been further criticized because of their emphasis on company 'commitment' rather than holding companies legally accountable to ensuring specific rights. Consequently, such patchwork self-regulation may result in 'enclave' social policy, governing select issues and groups of workers at specific points in their working lives. Such self-regulatory efforts may erode societal commitment to universal rights and entitlements in the process.

Business has established many self-regulatory mechanisms. While many support GHG, they are not without their disadvantages. Consequently, many health issues remain under the purview of public regulation. The commercial sector often considers that many of these domains are too important to leave to governments and intergovernmental organizations alone.

Commercial sector involvement in public governance

Where the commercial sector is not in a position to self-regulate, it will often seek to influence relevant public statutory regulation which might impact on its profits. Industry uses a number of mechanisms to exert its influence in relation to the content and process of the development of global public regulation and policy. Research has revealed efforts to:

1 Delay the introduction of international instruments (e.g. conventions, codes, agreements). For example, it is alleged that during the 1980s, the IFPMA delayed WHO efforts on a code of pharmaceutical marketing by arguing that it required time to implement its own voluntary code (Richter, 2001);

2 Block the adoption of an instrument. For example, the sugar industry provided the main opposition to the international dietary guidelines proposed by WHO in 2003;

3 Influence the content of an instrument. For example, tobacco companies lobbied at the national and international levels to secure changes to the text of the Framework Convention on Tobacco Control;

4 Challenge the credibility/validity of the instruments. For example, the Association of Infant Feeding Manufacturers has argued that a number of World Health Assembly resolutions which aim to interpret and update the International Code of Marketing Breastmilk Substitutes do not conform with the earlier resolution and are hence void;

5 Undermine the legitimacy and capacity of an international organization charged with negotiating an instrument. An enquiry into tobacco industry influence in WHO revealed that an elaborate, well financed, sophisticated and usually invisible global effort had been undertaken by the industry 'to divert attention from public health issues, to reduce budgets for the scientific and policy activities carried out by WHO, to pit other UN agencies against WHO, to convince developing countries that WHO's tobacco control programme was a "first world" agenda carried out at the expense of the developing world, to distort the results of important scientific studies, and to discredit WHO as an institution' (Zeltner et al., 2000);

6 Challenging the competence of a UN body to develop norms in a particular domain. For example, the food industry has tried to circumscribe the extent to which WHO can address obesity by proposing policies and regulations (Waxman, 2004).

The following case study illustrates one method that industry adopted to imprint its interests on global 'public' governance and the implications that this may have on health.

Susan Sell (2002) provides a detailed account of industry influence on the development of statutory rules which are virtually global in scope – the WTO TRIPS (Trade-Related Aspects of Intellectual Property Rights) Agreement. The impetus for global governance of IP arose from the recognition by certain industries that weak IP protection beyond the US resulted in widespread 'piracy' and a threat to their returns on investment in research and development (R&D). As a result, the CEOs of 12 US-based TNCs (representing firms in chemicals, information, entertainment, and pharmaceuticals), with an interest in world-wide protection of IP, established the Intellectual Property Committee (IPC). The Committee was formed just prior to the launch of the Uruguay Round of trade negotiations in 1987 which resulted in the establishment of the WTO and the adoption of its agreements.

The Committee operated as an informal network which sought global IP rights protection through international trade law. The Committee began by linking inadequate global protection of IP to US balance of payment deficits. Based on these economic arguments, and superior technical expertise, the IPC was able to alter the US administration's perceptions of its own interests and was thus able to win support of the US government for its aims. The IPC then sought to convince its industry allies in Canada, Japan and Europe of the logic of its

strategy of linking IP to international law and sought their support in lobbing their governments to support efforts to include IP protection in the Uruguay negotiations. In the interim,
the IPC hired a trade lawyer to draft an international IP treaty governing. The industry report
was adopted by the US administration as 'reflecting its views' and served as the negotiating
document in Uruguay. The IPC was able to position one of its members, the CEO of Pfizer, as
an advisor to the American delegation. Although the governments of India and Brazil
attempted to stall negotiations and drop IP from the round, economic sanctions imposed by
the US administration eventually undermined their opposition. As a result, agreement on
TRIPS was reached. According to the industry consultant who wrote the draft treaty, the 'IPC
got 95% of what it wanted' (Jaques Gorlin, quoted in Sell, 2003).

The TRIPS Agreement has the status of international law. As explained in Chapter
7, the WTO has responsibility to oversee the implementation of the Agreement and
has a particularly powerful enforcement mechanism. This case study provides an
example of relatively direct participation of industry in GHG.

Industry's success in governing IP from behind the scenes is likely to have profound implications for health. For example, the Agreement obliges countries that
had hitherto failed to protect product or process patents to make provisions for
doing so. The term on pharmaceutical patents is 20 years. Industry argues that
TRIPS will therefore ensure that firms continue to invest heavily in R&D to develop
innovative therapies. Critics point to the restrictions that the treaty places on the
use of generic drugs and the inevitable increase in the price of drugs as well as the
barriers to innovation that secrecy entails.

 Activity 13.6

> 1 Why does industry want binding, as opposed to voluntary, rules governing
>   intellectual property (IP)?
> 2 Why does industry seek global rules governing IP protection?
> 3 Why did the American administration support the goals of the Intellectual Property
>   Committee?
> 4 Why are global trade rules on IP significant for health?

 Feedback

> 1 Industry wanted binding measures so that all firms would have to comply. Voluntary
>   schemes often result in shallow and piecemeal compliance.
>
> 2 Industry wanted global rules as they did not wish for any countries to be in a position
>   to opt out.
>
> 3 The American administration is thought to have supported the aims of the IPC for a
>   number of reasons. First, the administration accepted industry's argument in relation to
>   the agreements improving the balance of payment deficit. Second, industry was able
>   to marshal considerable technical expertise as an input to the process. Third, these
>   industries provide considerable campaign finance to US political parties and spend
>   considerably to lobby on specific issues.
>
> 4 This case indicates that global trading rules governing IP will have positive implica-
>   tions for private finance of drug research and development (and by extension R&D

on any health-related technologies) and potentially negative implications in so far as widespread availability of the fruits of technological progress as ability to pay may be compromised.

Industry also attempts to shape the programmes of intergovernmental organizations. For example, documents released by the tobacco industry revealed ongoing efforts by the industry to influence WHO tobacco control programmes (Zeltner et al., 2000). Tobacco companies, their law firms and PR agencies hid evidence, subverted fact, employed ostensibly independent scientists and experts (secretly in pay) as well as the media and NGO-front organizations to influence the debate on tobacco. The expert enquiry into tobacco industry influence on WHO concluded that industry subversion of WHO tobacco control activities resulted in 'significant harm' but that the extent of which would be difficult to quantify.

Industry also targets the technical committees of intergovernmental organizations which routinely develop global norms and standards. For example, tobacco companies and their food company subsidiaries have employed the following strategies to exert influence on FAO/WHO food and nutrition policies developed in their respective expert committees (Hirschhorn, 2002):

- Philip Morris set up the International Tobacco Regulatory System to track a number of international organizations including FAO. This 'early warning system' was charged with drafting 'reasonable alternatives to new laws and regulations';
- Industry funded the 'International Council on Smoking Issues'. The Council monitored all international organizations based in Europe. So as to conceal the true identity and purpose of the Council, it used a third-party, PR firm which made requests in its name only;
- Industry 'positioned' experts on various FAO/WHO regulatory committees. As direct industry representation would be suspect, ostensibly independent experts were fielded but their conflicts of interest were not revealed. These 'independent' experts served, in industry's words, as industry's 'lawyers' and 'whole-hearted advocates';
- Industry was able to nominate such experts as a result of close relationships with staff in the FAO/WHO Secretariats. Hirschhorn argues that positioning is important because 'influence is exerted as much, perhaps more, by perusal persuasion as by scientific evidence'; and
- Industry provided financial support to sympathetic researchers to promote anti-regulatory ideology including attacks on WHO's dietary guidelines.

While Hirschhorn cannot marshal evidence to prove that industry was actually able to influence the content of specific regulations made by FAO/WHO committees, the evidence reveals that attempts were made in respect to sugars, pesticide use and residues, transfatty acids, additives and dietary guidelines. More revealing are industry claims that its strategies had indeed been effective. There is, therefore, substantial evidence that the commercial sector has actively sought to influence public regulation at the global level with a range of impacts on health.

Co-regulation

Co-regulation presents a third way between traditional public, statutory regulation and private self-regulation. It has arisen due to the inadequacies of public and private regulation. As you will recall, public statutory arrangements have been seen to be wanting in an era of globalization as state and intergovernmental capacity for regulation lags behind technological advances made by industry, suffers from jurisdictional constraints (i.e. national law doesn't apply in global space), and is often unaffordable and ineffective. Nonetheless, private self-regulation is often not always in the public's interest and thus a case remains for some external public control or hook on self-regulation. Co-regulation can be seen as public sector involvement in business self-regulation.

Co-regulation represents a bargain between public authorities and the private sector. The idea is that public and private sectors will negotiate on an agreed set of policy or regulatory objectives which are results-oriented. Subsequently, the private sector will take responsibility for implementation of the provisions. Monitoring compliance may remain a public responsibility or will be contracted out to a third party – sometimes an interested NGO. Indeed, co-regulatory initiatives often involve public, private and civil society organizations. The advent of co-regulation is relatively new, and there has been more formal experimentation with it at the national and regional levels. The Europe Union, for example, is experimenting with co-regulation particularly with respect to the Internet, journalism and e-commerce. The UN's Global Compact with industry might be viewed as a form of co-regulation as are many of the myriad of global public-private partnerships (PPPs) (Buse, 2004).

Global public-private health partnerships focus on different aspects of global health, including R&D for neglected diseases (e.g. International AIDS Vaccine Alliance), improving access to existing products through price discounting or donations (e.g. Mectizan Donation Program), raising additional resources for specific diseases (e.g. Global Fund for AIDS, TB and Malaria), or simply improved coordination of multiple actors (e.g. STOP TB). Such partnerships take a variety of organizational forms: as new institutions (e.g. the Medicines for Malaria Venture); or hosted by multilateral organizations (e.g. Roll Back Malaria in WHO); or hosted by international NGOs (e.g. Malaria Vaccine Initiative at PATH). Yet all of these PPP share four common features: actors from the private and public sectors work towards a shared goal; an explicit division of labour is agreed; all parties share in risks and benefits; and some form of shared or joint decision-making guides action.

While it is possible to characterize firm's aims with respect to PPP as simply philanthropic, placing them in the category of corporate social responsibility, or alternatively as vehicles designed to influence public sector governance, it is equally possible to conceive of PPPs as co-regulatory arrangements. First, partnerships are hybrid organizations which are neither pure public nor pure private in that there is some attempt to develop systems of rule in which both public and private actors have a voice in decision making. Second, PPPs govern substantive issue areas. For example, one analysis of PPPs found that most self-report the development of technical norms and standards in areas which had earlier been the preserve of public organizations (Buse, 2004).

Global health PPPs have had considerable impact in raising awareness, commitment and resources for specific communicable diseases and in accelerating progress, fostering R&D and reducing commodity prices. Yet there has been considerable controversy surrounding partnership as public and private interests do not always coincide and partnerships are often viewed as attempting to 'roll back' the welfare state.

 Activity 13.7

Make lists of the risks to the UN and to commercial actors of entering into partnership.

 Feedback

Your lists may have included the following:

Risks to private sector

- partnership with the UN may slow down and politicize decision making;
- waxing and waning commitment from public officials who come and go;
- high transaction costs;
- benefits incommensurate with costs;
- partners may disclosure proprietary or confidential information; and
- failure may damage to reputation.

Risks to UN

- participation of private sector in decision making may result in conflict of interest or undue influence;
- UN may become more accountable to private partners than member states;
- restrictions may be placed on disclosure of information and thus undermine transparency;
- attention to partnership activities may displace UN priorities;
- high transaction costs;
- benefits incommensurate with costs;
- association with disreputable firms may damage reputation; and
- confer unfair advantage on partner companies over competitors.

Summary

This chapter has provided an overview of the involvement of the commercial sector in GHG. You learned that this sector assumes many guises and that there are many ways that it attempts to 'steer' global health so as to pursue its financial interests. It is helpful to differentiate between self-regulation, influencing public-regulation, and co-regulation.

The purpose of a commercial organization is to generate profits and all activities of firms must be supported by a business case. It would be naïve to hope that the public interest and the pursuit of profit always coincide. Certainly many efforts by the private sector to engage in GHG are beneficial to public health, however, often trade-offs between profits and public health arise. Where these arise there are good grounds, from a public health perspective, for public regulation. Yet the extent to which the public sector, either nationally or internationally, is in a position to intervene is challenged both by increasing economic globalization and the ideology that underpins it.

References

Buse K (2004) 'Governing Public-Private Infectious Disease Partnerships'. *Brown Journal of World Affairs*. 10(2): 225–42.

Cattaui MS (1998) 'Business partnership forged on a global economy'. *ICC Press Release*. 6 February. Paris.

GIIC (1996) *Healthcare and Telemedicine*. Global Information Infrastructure Commission. www.giic.org/paper/policy/phealth.asp accessed 9 August 2004.

Hirschhorn N (2002) *How the tobacco and food industries and their allies tried to exert undue influence over FAO/WHO food and nutrition policies*. Unpublished. New Haven, CT.

Muggli ME, Hurt RD and Repace J (2004) 'The tobacco industry's political efforts to derail the EPA report on ETS'. *American Journal of Preventive Medicine*, 26(2): 167–77.

Richter J (2001) *Holding Corporations Accountable: Corporate conduct, international codes, and citizen action*. London: Zed Books.

Sell S (2003) *Private Power, Public Law: The Globalization of Intellectual Property*. Cambridge: Cambridge University Press.

Waxman HA (2004) 'Politics of international health in the Bush administration'. *Development*, 47(2): 24–8.

Zeltner T, Kessler DA, Martiny A and Randera F (2000) *Tobacco company strategies to undermine tobacco control activities at the World Health Organization*. Report of the Committee of Experts on Tobacco Industry Documents. Geneva: WHO.

Health and an emerging global civil society

Overview

In this final chapter you will learn about definitions of civil society, what is now known as global civil society, and the role of civil society organizations in health. You will then learn about the roles CSOs can and do play in promoting democracy and good global governance and how CSOs are involved in a wide range of activities at the global level. Finally you will see ways in which their legitimacy and accountability to undertake those roles can be enhanced.

Learning objectives

After working through this chapter, you should be able to:

- **understand what is meant by the term civil society and recognize the diverse character of CSOs**
- **assess the significance of developments in global civil society in response to broader global change**
- **discuss the multiple roles of CSOs in health governance**
- **consider the implications of the expanding role of CSOs in global governance for democracy, legitimacy and accountability.**

Key terms

Global civil society A sphere of ideas, values, institutions, organizations, networks and individuals located between the family, the state and the market, and operating beyond the confines of national societies, polities and economies.

Civil society – what is it?

 Activity 14.1

Make a list of some of the civil society initiatives that have influenced health that you are aware of.

Feedback

You may have thought of the usual suspects such as Médecins Sans Frontières. The health of individuals is produced across many sectors – potentially many different types of CSOs may therefore make a contribution. Historically, civil society initiatives have helped health in the past. It is important not to forget informal associations of individuals – such as home-based carers or women's credit groups – whose benefit to health can be enormous but which often goes largely unrecognized.

'Developments over the last two centuries demonstrate a pattern of governments reluctantly and sometimes hesitatingly following a trail blazed by NGOs'. (Weiss, 1999)

'. . . the NGO movement . . . is simply the analogue of the Western missionary movements of the past, which carried the gospel to the rest of the world and sought in this way to promote truth, salvation, and goodness'. (Anderson and Rieff, 2004)

You may have an instinctive view of what civil society means, and will doubtless think of the many big non-governmental organizations (NGOs) such as Oxfam, Greenpeace and Médecins Sans Frontières whose high-profile aid and campaigning work is often seen on our television screens. You may also be disposed to agree with the opinion of Thomas Weiss and his remarks about the 'trail-blazing' role that they play.

Others may be more sceptical and attracted instead to the challenges of Kenneth Anderson and David Rieff. Who are these NGOs to lecture on the values of human rights and democracy to the rest of the world? To whom are *they* accountable?

A recent United Nations (UN) publication defines civil society as follows:

'associations of citizens (outside their families, friends and businesses) entered into voluntarily to advance their interests, ideas and ideologies. The term does not include profit-making activity (the private sector) or governing (the public sector)'. (UN, 2004).

This is a broad definition. It might include, for example, the following types of organizations: labour unions, faith-based groups, professional associations, academic and research institutions, human rights networks, consumer rights coalitions, social movements, social and sports clubs, philanthropic foundations, and other forms of 'associational life', both formal and informal (UNDP, 1997). The mafia, choirs and dog-breeding clubs might be considered just as much a part of civil society as Amnesty International.

The same UN publication defines NGOs somewhat differently.

'All organisations . . . that are not central governments and were not created by intergovernmental decision, including associations of businesses, parliamentarians and local authorities.'

The authors – a distinguished international panel of experts – note the 'considerable confusion' surrounding the use of the term NGO. Most of us do identify them with organizations in the mould of Oxfam (more precisely called *public-benefit*

NGOs because they are set up to provide a benefit through advocacy or services to the public at large). We do not tend to think of other organizations, such as the International Federation of Pharmaceutical Manufacturers' Associations or the Inter-Parliamentary Union – a global federation of parliaments – as being in the same category.

 Activity 14.2

Compare the definitions of civil society and NGOs in the UN report. Do you think the report is making a useful distinction? Give reasons for your answer.

 Feedback

The UN makes an implicit distinction between the relatively formal structure of NGOs and the more amorphous 'informal' world of dense interconnections that constitutes civil society. This is a useful reminder of the breadth of civil society. Nevertheless, there are confusions: for example, the definition of civil society rules out 'profit-making activity'; the NGO definition does not. This lack of clarity may make distinctions between those NGOs who represent business and those who work for the 'public benefit' more difficult for the UN to operationalize in its day-to-day work.

The definitions provided by the UN may themselves cause 'considerable confusion'. But perhaps this is inevitable. In reality, there can often be no clear distinctions made between the state, civil society, and markets and the private-for-profit sector. Many CSOs depend for a large proportion of their income on state support, and others are heavily dependent on their business activities, such as sales of goods or consultancy fees. Market pressures also shape the way CSOs behave – for example, forcing them to act in a more 'business-like' way to attract investment in the market for international aid. As John Keane notes, market forces produce considerable inequalities between CSOs: Greenpeace with an annual budget of US$100 million and the World Wildlife Fund with US$170 million are very much bigger than the vast majority of CSOs and even wealthier than the United Nations Environment Programme.

Governments have also been involved in the creation of civil society groups, through funding and even direct political control. The creation of 'GONGOs' (government owned NGOs) is often associated with political patronage, involving the creation of charitable bodies run by and often benefiting government supporters with little benefit to the public. Government support to service provision NGOs as a way of managing declines in public expenditure and encouraging societal self-reliance is also well-known. However, it should be noted that a government may well promote the emergence of CSOs in order to 'make a rod for its own back', by setting up organizations which can monitor its performance and mobilize groups of people to demand accountability.

In this chapter the term civil society organizations is used in the broad sense outlined in the UN definition (incorporating NGOs as well), although we recognize that there may be important instances when the categories have to be made clearer.

For example, many commentators have protested about the elision of differences between *public*-interest CSOs and *private*- (or *mutual*)-interest ones in operational definitions of civil society organizations. Research indicates that around half of the bodies registered as CSOs at the UN are affiliated with business interests in some way. 'Corporations have been creating PR "front" organizations and pseudo-grassroots or "Astroturf" groups and networks that outsiders can find difficult to distinguish from genuine activist citizens groups', the policy-analyst Judith Richter has observed. A lack of ability to distinguish between the categories could affect decision-making abilities, allowing private-interest CSOs to mask a hidden, commercial agenda with a public face, in their interactions with UN (and other) bodies. Such issues are particularly important in the field of health, where commercial interests are strong. We return to them below.

Civil society and health

Civil society has often played a key role in promoting health at the national level: the history of the UK is replete with examples of action by groups of individual citizens to provide health facilities to the indigent and needy – today's UK National Health Service was forged from the patchwork of public and private action which made up the pre-1948 health service. Powerful associations – such as the Royal College of Physicians of London – have existed since the sixteenth century to represent the interests of their members and to regulate their professions. Tackling the causes of ill-health through the provision of charity to the destitute in the form of financial support and employment opportunities also has a long history. The UK government still sees civil society as a key player in its overall health policy – and it continues to support it, for example by providing statutory funding to large charities undertaking research or service provision for particular conditions. The story is the same in many other parts of the world, with private non-profit organizations (often religious in nature) providing large parts of health services in many low-income countries.

Civil society has also had an increasing influence on international health policy. During the 1970s, for example, health-related CSOs played an influential role in the development of primary health care as an international policy. Innovative projects such as Gonoshasthaya Kendra (the People's Health Centre) in Bangladesh, greatly influenced the shift towards a more politicized, social definition of health. Another significant player during this period was the International Baby Food Action Network (IBFAN) which lobbied successfully for the adoption of the International Code on the Marketing of Breastmilk Substitutes by the World Health Assembly in 1981.

Yet it is also true that many aspects of civil society important for sustaining health are terribly under-researched, especially in the developing world, and the focus on large public-interest CSOs and prominent networks is in some sense diverting our attention from the large numbers of self-help activities and other forms of associational life such as hometown associations, lineages, age-sets, elders' committees, home-based carers' associations and women's credit groups (Lewis, 2002). More research certainly needs to be done into the activities of these groups and their particular interests and values – which will vary enormously. It is important to remember their existence when we think about the potential involvement of civil society in global health governance later in this chapter.

Table 14.1 categorizes civil society action in health by geographical influence (local, national, international) and direction of benefit (mutual- or private- versus public-benefit). Note that the category boundaries are not solid – some organizations have multiple roles – for example, although they may be providing a service for their members they may also play a wider 'public-benefit' role by providing information or services to the population at large. A national level organization may have considerable international influence even if it doesn't have branches in other countries. The blurring of distinctions in the table between mutual-benefit and private-benefit may also be controversial for some.

Table 14.1 Categorization of civil society actions in health

	Mutual-/Private-benefit	Public-benefit
International	• World Medical Association • International Federation of Pharmaceutical Manufacturers' Associations	• Médecins Sans Frontières • MERLIN • Amnesty International
National	• UK Royal College of Nursing • British Medical Association	• Cancer Research (UK) • Gonoshasthaya Kendra (Bangladesh) • Treatment Action Campaign (South Africa)
Local	• Community-level health insurance schemes	• Local charities

Source: Adapted from Thomas 1992.

 Activity 14.3

Can you think of other organizations to add to Table 14.1?

 Feedback

Mutual-Private-benefit International: International Council of Nurses, International Union of Immunological Societies.

Mutual-Private-benefit National: Health Visitors Association; timebanks.

Mutual-Private-benefit Local: buddy schemes for HIV patients

Public-benefit International: Corporate Accountability International

Public-benefit National: The Aids Support Organization (TASO), Uganda; Consumers Association UK; National Heart Forum, UK

Global civil society

IBFAN is a good example of a new category of civil society groups that has emerged strongly over the last 20 to 30 years – *global* civil society. Kaldor et al. (2004) describe this as

> 'a sphere of ideas, values, institutions, organisations, networks and individuals located *between* the family, the state, and the market, and operating *beyond* the confines of national societies, polities and economies.'

The emergence of global civil society has been in part prompted by changes in communication and other technologies – the compression of space and time accompanying globalization you saw in Chapter 1 – which has allowed greater communication and networking between countries. However, global civil society has also emerged *in reaction* to the process of globalization – the discovery that many issues are cross-border and non-territorial in nature, such as the fight against infectious diseases, or the struggle for women's rights; and the perceived negative influence of unaccountable global corporations and multilateral bodies such as the International Monetary Fund and World Bank, which are under the control of no individual government.

Mention should also be made of money. CSOs, particularly from Europe, have strengthened and multiplied their international links through funding partner organizations across the developing world, increasing the density of 'global civil society' (Anheier et al., 2001). Governmental donors and philanthropic agencies (such as the Rockerfeller Foundation) have also been busy financing global networks on particular themes.

As a result of all these trends, there has been an explosion in numbers of 'international non-governmental organizations' (INGOs) over the last decade. By 2001, INGOs numbered around 13,000, up by a quarter since 1990 (Anheier et al., 2001).

The most visible part of global civil society is perhaps the strong growth of these 'transnational advocacy networks', and their existence has led to much discussion and debate. They are not new. The campaign to abolish slavery in the early nineteenth century was transnational in character, as have been various protests and campaigns against war in the twentieth century and the campaign against the Apartheid regime in South Africa during the 1970s and 1980s. However, the advocacy networks now appear to be greater in number and are receiving more attention and study than ever before. Commentators have noted how the 'voluntary, reciprocal, and horizontal patterns of communication and exchange' which characterize them results in effective networks with 'fluid and open relations among committed and knowledgeable actors working in specialized issue areas' (Keck and Sikkink, 1998). They can be devastatingly effective. Recent worldwide campaigns against the Multilateral Agreement on Investment and third world debt, as well as for the rights of people living with HIV/AIDS are especially prominent examples of the genre.

Alarm has grown among governments and in the boardrooms of international corporations at the emergence of what has been dubbed the 'NGO swarm' with no 'central leadership or command-structure ... multi-headed, impossible to decapitate' (*The Economist*, 1999). As a result of this high-profile activity, concern is now often expressed about to whom the 'swarm' is accountable and from whence it gains it legitimacy. Commentators such as Anderson and Rieff argue that global civil society represents a new kind of imperialism in the sphere of values. They raise key questions about civil society's relationship with democracy, to which we turn below.

The development of an advocacy community around HIV/AIDS has been usefully analysed by Seckinelgen (2002), and Table 14.2 shows the way in which it has developed over the past two decades, building from local and nationally based coalitions of people concerned with patients' needs into a transnational grouping of strong organizations undertaking research, lobbying and campaigning. As in the case of IBFAN, groups have been able to push the issue of HIV/AIDS to the top of the agenda not only because of the vigorous work of organizations and individuals linked across many countries, but also because of the increasing efforts on the part of governments to deal with this issue at the international level, through global summits and the setting up of a global body to respond to the problem, in this case UNAIDS. In this respect, governmental and non-governmental efforts have, to some extent, been synergistic.

Table 14.2 The globalization of the civil society response to HIV/AIDS

1980s————————————→	1990s————————————→	2000+
Provision	Campaigns and lobbying	Internationalization
Patients' groups – Locality-based structures providing care and support in developed and developing countries; church-based groups – More formal structures such as Terence Higgins Trust in UK; TASO in Uganda; PDA in Thailand	Treatment activism – ACT-UP founded in late 1980s in USA; Treatment Action Campaign in South Africa started in 1990s – Engagement with scientists/medical profession	Provoked by: – Involvement of UN agencies (e.g. WHO/UNAIDS/World Bank) – International conferences and summits – International solidarity between CSOs working on HIV/AIDS and the growth of global civil society

Source: Adapted from Seckinelgin (2002).

Civil society, democracy and global governance

'Civil society organisations are . . . the glory of democratic societies, but they are not the electoral institutions of democracy'. (Anderson and Rieff, 2004: 30)

Our positive understanding of the role of civil society has been formed by some of the key events of the late-twentieth century, most notably the Velvet Revolutions against Communism in Eastern Europe in the late-1980s, where civil action – nurtured through years of underground activity – peacefully crushed dictatorship after dictatorship. International agencies and donor countries have also highlighted the role that civil society can play in democratization and have funded projects to boost its presence across the developing world.

Authors such as Anderson and Rieff show that civil society can play an important role in the democratic process within the context of the nation-state through the way in which it represents a disparate array of voices outside the sphere of parliamentary democracy. Civil society can strengthen people's claims on the state and voice opinions which may not otherwise be voiced: it strengthens democracy. Yet it does not seek to supplant the procedures of democracy (elections, parliament, the law). Democratically elected politicians, these authors argue, *not* civil society, represent the people.

At the global level, however, there is no set of democratically elected institutions. But increasingly – as demonstrated throughout this volume – decisions which affect people's everyday lives are being taken at the global as well as at the national level. Anderson and Rieff argue that this democratic deficit is being filled by a global civil society which stakes a claim to be representative of the people of the world and to 'intermediate' between them and unaccountable global institutions. The authors note that this raises important questions about who global civil society really does represent; and they imply that the lack of procedural democracy at the global level undermines the legitimacy of such a 'representation' role for global civil society. They complain that global civil society today is acting like the missionaries of old – exporting the gospel (of human rights) to the (former) colonial lands; universalizing *one* set of values over the multiple and clashing values which would necessarily be represented if democratic institutions existed at the global level.

However, if globalization is leading to fewer and fewer policy decisions being taken at the national level, then surely it is right, and strengthens democracy, for the organizations and networks of global civil society to ensure that the global institutions that take those decisions are made more accountable. While there is no global parliament it remains relevant to draw on another important distinction between the procedures of democracy (elections, parliaments, etc) and the *substance* of democracy, which is surely concerned with the extent to which individual citizens can influence the decisions that affect their lives (Kaldor et al., 2004). Commentators who take this view accuse writers like Anderson and Rieff of being 'nostalgic for an era of national simplicities' (Kaldor et al., 2004: 16), and argue that global civil society – however imperfect in its representivity – can play a key role in the democratization of global institutions and processes.

We should pause here to consider more deeply this putative relationship between civil society and democracy, which all sides seem to agree on. Given the diversity of civil society outlined at the beginning of this chapter – remember the dog-breeders and the mafia – can we really say that there is a necessary relationship between the existence of one and the existence of the other? Of course not. But likewise it would be foolish to deny that civil society has not played an important role in democracy – either by supporting it, being neutral towards it (the dog-breeders), or undermining it (the mafia). The relationship must be assessed on a case-by-case basis. Perhaps, as Hilary Wainright argues, it is best to say that civil society action has the *potential* to deepen democracy.

Activity 14.4

What is your view on the opinions put forward by Anderson and Rieff? Do you agree with them?

Feedback

Anderson and Rieff could be accused, not only of nostalgia but also of underestimating the diversity of civil society. Those on the other side of the debate might be equally be said to be exaggerating its diversity and potential for deepening democracy! It's a matter of opinion. There is also a key question – especially in relation to international development issues – of the balance of power between NGOs and Southern governments.

Returning to our discussion of the role of global civil society, both sides of this debate would probably agree that in the end the most pertinent issue is to find ways of ensuring that there is some degree of accountability and representativeness among the multiplicity of players who make up global civil society. Michael Edwards (2000) in his book *NGO Rights and Responsibilities* proposes a three-point 'New Deal' between governments and civil society to address concerns:

Firstly, there need to be formal structures where CSO voices can be heard – without pretending that they can substitute for governments. Regular global forums where CSOs can participate and debate global governance issues with decision makers might be one method.

Secondly, CSOs should be able to participate in global governance in return for agreeing to a set of minimal standards on integrity and performance. Self-regulation would be the key, with international bodies also continuing with their assessments of CSOs' suitably to liaise with them.

Thirdly, the playing field needs to be levelled to ensure that there is greater access and representation for Southern governments and CSOs.

CSOs have generally welcomed such proposals, subject to two caveats – firstly, standards should not stop CSOs from raising uncomfortable questions with the governments and global institutions. And secondly, they are wary about whether institutions of global governance will actually become more welcoming and less exclusionary in return for CSO self regulation.

A final key point raised by CSOs is how private- or commercial-interest CSOs are to be dealt with by international agencies. There have been major problems in this area in the past. Key policy making committees in institutions such as WHO have been packed with representatives of commercial companies, sometimes working for 'CSOs', and with the same rights as public-benefit CSOs. The failure of global institutions to make a distinction between public- and commercial-interest CSOs has been strongly protested.

Global health governance and the roles of civil society

Table 14.3 shows some of the bodies involved in performing and influencing global health governance.

Clearly, many organizations with supra-national influence are taking decisions which will affect people's health worldwide. Equally clearly, civil society groups

Table 14.3 Fragments of the global health governance mosaic

Body	Role
World Health Organization	Global normative and standard setting agency for health
UNAIDS	The leading agency for worldwide action against HIV/AIDS, its purpose is to lead, strengthen and support an expanded response to the epidemic
UNICEF	Lead international agency for children's issues with a particular focus on education and health
G7	2000 Summit of G7 leaders led to Okinawa summit on infectious diseases; economic policy decisions indirectly affect the health of billions
World Trade Organization	Trade agreements (on issues such as agriculture, intellectual property rights, trade in services and competition) made at the World Trade Organization have direct and indirect impact on health and health services worldwide
International Labour Office	Promotes workers' health; studies the impact on workers of health sector reform
World Summit on Population and Development (Cairo, 1994)	Set the agenda for reproductive health policy
World Bank	1993 World Development Report 'Investing in Health' set the global health policy agenda for the 1990s
International Monetary Fund	Sets restrictive limits on fiscal deficits in low-income countries, blamed for decline in health services in the least developed countries over the last 20 years
Organization for Economic Co-operation and Development	Formulated the International Development Targets (re-formulated as the Millennium Development Goals by the UN General Assembly), now the primary goals for aid donors and recipients
European Union	Directorate for trade responsible for negotiating position on public health in World Trade Organization agreements
US Institutes of Medicine	1997 report defining HIV/AIDS and other infectious diseases as a foreign policy issue widely credited for ensuring US administration saw the problem of infectious diseases as important
US Congress/American CSOs	CSOs lobbied US Congress to ensure that the World Bank was disallowed from promoting user fees for primary health and education services as part of its loan conditions
Health Action International, Treatment Action Campaign, Oxfam, Médecins Sans Frontières, and other Southern and Northern CSOs	Lobbied national and international trade representatives to insert public health clause into agreement at the 2001 World Trade Organization Summit at Doha (so-called 'Doha declaration')

will be attempting to influence these organizations. What then are the roles that civil society can play in global health governance? What pitfalls do they face when playing these roles? And how can some of the issues raised by Michael Edwards be dealt with?

Role 1: Representing 'the voice of the people'

From our previous discussion this is clearly a controversial proposition, and one that it is important to subject to scrutiny. Nevertheless many actors in health do – implicitly or explicitly – make this claim, simply by presenting their concerns to national and global institutions. One example of an explicit claim is the People's Health Movement.

The establishment and growth of the People's Health Movement (PHM), following the People's Health Assembly held in December 2000, is a good example of an emerging player in global civil society. The PHM is a transnational network, originally conceived of by a group of organizations with membership spread across the world (including Consumers International, Health Action International Asia-Pacific and Women's Global Network on Reproductive Rights) and which now has emerging regional bases in South Asia, Latin America, sub-Saharan Africa, Europe and North America. The Movement's first Assembly in Bangladesh was attended by over 1,400 people from around 90 countries. The Movement argues that urgent attention is required to address both the underlying causes of ill-health, such as poverty, and the need to create more equitable and sustainable health systems.

The PHM has broad and ambitious goals: first, to re-establish health and equitable development as top priorities in local, national and international policy making, and second, to promote comprehensive primary health care as the strategy to achieve these priorities. In order to do this it both draws on and supports people's movements in their struggles to build long-term and sustainable solutions to health problems (www.phmovement.org). The PHM emphasizes increasing the participation of local people in global health debates – on hearing the 'voices of the unheard'.

The PHM is run by a global coordinating committee, made up primarily of members of the founding CSOs and, since the Assembly, of elected regional representatives. On a day-to-day basis, the secretariat in Bangalore makes administrative decisions and puts forward strategic campaigning priorities such as the recent million-signature campaign for 'Health for All', although anyone is welcome to do so.

Activity 14.5

Use the information provided above to establish the core values and interests that the PHM appears to represent. Has the PHM has undertaken appropriate actions to ensure its legitimacy and accountability?

Feedback

- There is evidence from the organizational composition of PHM (it is a network of networks); from the widespread support for its first Assembly; and from the developing regional infrastructure that the Movement has some degree of accountability.

- Questions of leadership and representation have been important within PHM from its inception. While it is still a developing movement, and its internal governance is liable to change, an extensive evaluation exercise found broad satisfaction among participants regarding such issues.
- The complex structure of PHM's governance highlights the extent to which the movement has sought to reconcile tensions between the commitment to democracy and the need for leadership and coordination. Organized around interacting circles based on regional and issue-based representation as well as Secretarial support, this structure seeks to reflect the diversity within PHM.

Role 2: Advocacy and lobbying

Broadly speaking there are two approaches to CSO advocacy: the first is a confrontational approach which deploys powerful counter-narratives against selected institutions, governments and other actors in development processes and which helps to dislodge entrenched policy positions – the Jubilee 2000 campaign on international debt is a good example of this type of pressure. A second approach is more participatory and consensual and emphasizes developing institutions where dialogue about policy issues can take place (Harper, 2001). Major successes have been achieved over the years in pushing international health debates forward, through various combinations of these two strategies. Campaigns on infant feeding and drug pricing are two prominent examples. However, it is also the case that CSO campaigns and lobbying can be too focused on a single entry point in socio-economic processes, creating change on a particular subject but not dealing with the underlying issues (Krut, 1997). Campaigns on banning child labour, for instance, have often had this charge levelled at them particularly as prohibiting children's ability to work can push households into greater hardship and children into more hazardous employment, such as sex work (Chapman, 2001).

Role 3: Research and policy analysis

Research and policy analysis programmes in health have been initiated by a range of CSOs, with frequent sharing of information and research via advocacy networks. Through partnerships and advocacy networks, the experience of CSOs in the South has been frequently used to highlight local impacts of global policy. A benefit of CSO research may be a willingness to fund and explore issues not confronted by academics and more mainstream research funding institutions. On the other hand, a lack of capacity (financial and human) for proper research may lead to low standards and leave the CSO open to accusations of 'gathering anecdotes'.

Role 4: Watchdog

The role of 'watchdog' or counterweight, is slightly different than advocacy and clearly associated with research and analysis. CSOs would position themselves to ask 'difficult and challenging questions'. Often this comes in the form of reports on the monitoring of codes and standards, or in press releases or short reports on, for example, compliance with international development goals. Sometimes, this counterweight role has become more formalized, for example with the establishment of separate organizations which perform a 'watchdog' role on specific international institutions. A notable example is the Bretton Woods Project in the United Kingdom, conceived by a network of British CSOs in the mid-1990s to monitor the IMF and the World Bank but which operates as an independent organization. The Project provides information to CSOs, governments and journalists and citizens from around the world on the full-breadth of IMF and World Bank activities. In the health sector IBFAN, through its six regional coordinating offices, works closely with groups in 90 countries in monitoring the actions of the baby-foods industry and their adherence to the International Code on the Marketing of Breastmilk Substitutes.

Again, concerns about legitimacy and accountability, especially with regard to Southern partners, applies to watchdogs and they have a particular duty to spread information to 'voiceless' parts of civil society as well as to do their best to bring information from the grassroots to the attention of policy makers. Paul Nelson argues that there is also a need for watchdogs in North and South working on similar issues to collaborate closely, in order to gain a better understanding of common needs and priorities.

Role 5: Communication

CSOs have played an important role in ensuring greater transparency in the policy process, through information-sharing and broadcasting policy decisions. Their ability to do this has been magnified by technological advances and especially the advent of the Internet. However, this spreading of knowledge needs to reach Southern and grassroots partners instead of it just circulating among Northern colleagues, in order to fully enable participation in global health governance.

Role 6: Involvement in 'horizontal' governance mechanisms

'Producing health' is a multi-sectoral activity. Consequently, responsibility for global governance in health is dispersed across a number of agencies, resulting in the inevitable problems of coordination and overlapping mandates. WHO, UNICEF, UNAIDS, UNFPA, UNDP, the ILO and the World Bank are all involved in health issues, along with a host of regional actors and complemented by a battery of international human rights law. As a complement to this diversity of international agencies, CSOs not specifically dedicated to health could be encouraged to broaden their involvement with global health governance issues. For example, better alliances with human rights groups (Amnesty, Human Rights Watch, etc), the international financial and trade institution-watch groups, labour rights groups and women's rights groups could link key global health issues into wider efforts toward sustainable development. WHO could also perform a valuable task by providing a coordination or liaison role between the spectrum of global institutions and CSOs involved in international health. This role would be particularly important in ensuring complementarity in actions by pooling resources, maximizing outcomes, and preventing duplication and fragmentation. However, there is a danger that CSO efforts to network horizontally will be lost without a parallel commitment on the part of international institutions to coordinate activities at the same time.

Role 7: Involvement in multi-level governance

Having an impact on global governance also requires engaging with different levels of governance, including interaction with national governments where CSOs are based. Inclusion as part of a governmental delegation to an international conference may enhance CSO leverage in influencing policy at the global level. The overall aim of multi-level governance should be to enhance national responsiveness to global health needs and global responsiveness to local health needs. However, CSO participation on governmental delegations, unless carefully managed, can lead to CSOs feeling co-opted and restrict their range of advocacy positions. There is also a danger that inequalities will develop between 'privileged' CSOs on governmental delegations and 'underprivileged' CSOs outside.

Role 8: Horizontal and vertical networking

Networking with member organizations, other CSOs and non-state actors (horizontal networking), and government and multilateral agencies (vertical networking) has contributed significantly to changing or modifying global agendas. Networking and the dispersal of information has been improved both by the existence of global fora (such as the UN conferences) around which activists can mobilize (and actually meet at) and, most dramatically over the last decade, by use of the Internet. Women's transnational networks demonstrated their valuable strategic role in the run-up both to the UN Conference on Human Rights held in Vienna in 1993 and at the International Conference on Population and Development in Cairo. Involvement in such networks serves to multiply the impact of their collective views on global health policy.

Role 9: Build capacity of civil society organizations

Northern CSOs frequently play an important role in overcoming the under-representation of Southern/grassroots CSOs by transferring resources to strengthen these organizations, as well as contacts and information. However, where capacity is already strong, direct financial support to Southern CSOs to prepare for and attend global meetings, for example, may be preferable to support for organizational development.

Role 10: CSOs collaborate with global health institutions in designing and implementing promotion, prevention and control programmes

CSOs around the world play an important role in delivering health interventions – in some parts of the world, especially in sub-Saharan Africa, they perform a majority of health service functions. In addition, there is some evidence to show that they can be effective at reaching poorer and marginalized groups missed by governments, although this is a proposition that certainly does not hold universally, with studies showing that poor people have often not been reached by CSO services or that CSOs contribute to inequitable coverage and fragmentation. Nevertheless, while CSOs hold such a dominant service provider position in some countries, their opinions should, as a matter of course, be sought by governments and international institutions engaging with health issues. They can bring a sense of reality to decision making and provide policy makers with examples of innovative ways of delivering health interventions. Care is needed, however, that unsustainable resource-intensive strategies do not overwhelm fragile and resource-poor government systems.

Summary

You have learnt about the diverse character of civil society organizations, assessed the significance of developments in global civil society in response to broad global changes and the multiple roles that CSOs occupy in health governance. Finally, you considered the implications of expanding the role of CSOs in global governance.

References

Anderson K and Rieff D (2004) 'Global Civil Society: a sceptical view'. In *Global Civil Society 2004/5* (Anheier H et al., eds). London: Sage.

Anheier H, Glasius M and Kaldor M (2001) 'Introducing global civil society'. In *Global Civil Society 2001* (Anheier H, Glasius M and Kaldor M, eds). Oxford: Oxford University Press.

Chapman J (2001) 'What makes international campaigns effective? Lessons from India and Ghana'. In *Global Citizen Action* (Edwards M and Gaventa J eds). London: Earthscan.

Economist, The (1999). The Non-Governmental Order: Will NGOs Democratise, or Merely Disrupt, Global Governance? 11–17 December. Available at http://www.globalpolicy.org/ngos/99role.htm (accessed 27 February 2005).

Edwards M (2000) 'Time to put the NGO house in order'. *Financial Times*, London 6 June. Available at http://fpc.org.uk/articles/77 (accessed 27 February 2005).

Harper C (2001) 'Do the facts matter? NGOs, research and international advocacy'. In *Global Citizen Action* (Edwards M and Gaventa J, eds). London: Earthscan.

Kaldor M et al. (2005) 'Introduction'. In *Global Civil Society 2005* (Anheier H et al., eds). London: Sage.

Keck M and Sikkink K (1998) *Activists beyond Borders. Advocacy networks in international politics.* Ithaca: Cornell University Press.

Krut R (1997) *Globalization and Civil Society: NGO Influence in International Decision-Making.* Discussion Paper No. 83, April 1997. Geneva: UNRISD. http://www.unrisd.org/engindex/publ/list/dp/dp83/toc.htm.

Lewis D (2002) 'Civil society in African contexts: reflections on the usefulness of a concept'. *Development and Change*, 33(4): 569–86.

Seckinelgin H (2002) 'Time to stop and think: HIV/AIDS, global civil society, and people's politics' in Glasius M, Kaldor M and Anheier H, eds, *Global Civil Society 2002*. Oxford: Oxford University Press. http://www.lse.ac.uk/Depts/global/Yearbook/PDF/PDF2002/GCS2002%20pages%20[05]%20.pdf.

Thomas, A. 'Non-governmental organisations and the limits to empowerment'. In, Wuyts et al., eds *Development Policy and Public Action*. Oxford University Press, 1992. Figure 5.3; 123.

UN (2004) *We the peoples: civil society, the United Nations and global governance: Report of the Panel of Eminent Persons on United Nations – Civil Society Relations*. New York: UN.

Weiss T (1999) *International NGOs, global governance, and social policy in the UN system*. GASPP Occasional Papers No. 3. Globalism and Social Policy Programme. http://www.stakes.fi/gaspp/occasional%20papers/gaspp3-1999-pdf.

Parts of this chapter were excerpted from Fustukian, S, Rowson M and Papineni, P, 'Global governance for health – the emerging role of civil society' (unpublished, 2003).

Glossary

Adaptation An action (or spontaneous change) that lessens the adverse impacts of GEC.

Anarchy The condition under which sovereign states interact with each other without recognizing any common, superior authority over their individual and collection actions.

Biodiversity The natural range of species (or intra-species genetic strains) within an ecosystem which provides a source of resilience, stability and productivity.

Carrying capacity The size of population that can be indefinitely supported by the natural resource base of the specified geographic area.

Civil society Associations of citizens (outside their families, friends and businesses) entered into voluntarily to advance their interests, ideas and ideologies.

Classical regime The international governance framework that developed in the first century of international health diplomacy.

Climate change Long-term change (over decades, centuries or millennia) in average meteorological conditions (such as temperature and rainfall).

Climate variability Shifts in climatic patterns that are relatively short-term (over years or decades) but that go beyond individual weather events.

Code of conduct Voluntary measure undertaken by a firm to impact upon some aspect of its business practice.

Compulsory license The permission given by a government to a third party to use or produce an invention without the consent of the patent holder.

Corporate social responsibility Industry supported measures whereby companies attempt to demonstrate responsible behaviour.

Corporation An association of stockholders which is regarded as an artificial person under most national laws. Ownership is marked by ease of transferability and stockholders have limited liability.

Cultural globalization The blurring of previously accepted boundaries which differentiated states, ethnicities and civil societies such that new spaces of daily life, new sources of cultural meaning, and new forms of social and political agency flow across national borders.

Dietary changes Changes in the type and mix of foods consumed.

Dimensions of global change The three types of changes – spatial, temporal and cognitive – taking place that characterize globalization.

Drug approval agencies National and international bodies that must approve the safety and efficacy of a drug before it can be used.

Dumping The placing of products in the international market at well below their production costs.

Economic globalization The process by which flows of goods and services, capital, labour or other means of production and exchange cross, and increasingly circumvent, national borders.

Emerging infection An infection that has newly appeared in a population, or has previously existed but is rapidly increasing in incidence or geographic range.

Food marketing The promotion of certain foods through the media and/or placement of vending machines in public places.

Food security The situation when all people, at all times, have physical, social and economic access to sufficient, safe and nutritious food that meets their dietary needs and food preferences for an active and healthy life.

Gender A socio-economic variable with which to analyse roles, responsibilities, constraints and opportunities of men and women.

Gender perspective A gender perspective tries to discern the impact of gender in terms of structural (legal and economic), social (education, health and religious) and cultural mother, leader, carer dimensions.

Generic drug A copy of a medicine produced once its patent protection expires and usually sold under its chemical rather than brand name.

Global civil society A sphere of ideas, values, institutions, organizations, networks and individuals located between the family, the state and the market, and operating beyond the confines of national societies, polities and economies.

Global economy An economy whereby production, exchange, and consumption are not linked to territorial distances but transcend national borders (transborder).

Global environmental change Large-scale human-induced changes in the Earth's natural environment in recent decades as a reflection of unprecedented impacts on the biosphere.

Global governance Governance among states (including intergovernmental organizations) and non-state actors (e.g. non-governmental organizations and multinational corporations).

Global health A health issue where the determinants circumvent, undermine or are oblivious to the territorial boundaries of states and, thus, beyond the capacity of individual countries to address through domestic institutions.

Global health governance Governance efforts among states and non-state actors for purposes of protecting and promoting human health.

Global health security The set of issues where global health and national security concerns overlap, including infectious disease epidemics and bioterrorism.

Global public goods for health Products or services connected to promoting or protecting health that exhibit a significant degree of non-rivalry and non-excludability in consumption across national boundaries and traditional regional groupings.

Global society The idea that globalization is leading to peoples being incorporated into a single world society.

Global village The concept that people are increasingly holding notions of society that combine micro-level (community, district, nationality) and macro-level (world) identities.

Globalization A set of global processes that are changing the nature of human interaction across a wide range of social spheres including the economic, political, cultural and environmental.

Governance The process of governing, or of controlling, managing, or regulating the affairs of some entity.

Government The institutions and procedures for making and enforcing rules and other collective decisions. A narrower concept.

Horizontal governance Governance by means of cooperation between sovereign states.

Human right to health The right of individuals to the highest attainable standard of health.

Human security The protection of individual life and well-being from threats.

Industry Groups of firms closely related by use of similar technology of production or high level of substitutability of products.

Intellectual property Creations of the mind, including inventions, literary and artistic works, and symbols, names, images and designs. It is of two types: industrial (e.g. patents and trademarks) and copyright (e.g. musical).

International economy An economy whereby production, exchange and consumption take place across national borders (crossborder) between entities located in two or more countries.

International governance The process of governing the relations between states that involves only the states as legitimate actors.

International law The body of rules that regulates the interactions of states and, in certain situations, the relationships between individuals and the state.

Medicalization The tendency for a range of problems to be defined as medical and therefore are subject to the influence and control of medicine.

Most favoured nation principle In a trade agreement between two countries, if either party to the treaty grants a favour (usually a tariff reduction) to a third country, the other party to the treaty will be granted the same favour.

National governance Governance that takes place within a single sovereign state.

National security The defence of the state against military and other types of serious threats to the state's survival and well-being.

Neo-Westphalian governance The return of Westphalian governance characteristics in health policy in the 1990s and early 2000s.

Non tariff barrier Barriers to trade that are either quota or quantitative restrictions deliberately designed to protect domestic industries or internal taxes, administrative requirements, health and sanitary regulations and government procurement policies that are not necessarily intended to restrict trade.

Parallel import The importation of a product without the approval of the owner of patent or trademark or copyright.

Patent A formal licence that an invention cannot be copied in the jurisdiction for which it is applied.

Population at risk A population subgroup that is more likely to be exposed or is more sensitive to an infection than is the general population.

Post-Westphalian governance The governance framework that developed in international health policy after the Second World War under the influence of the World Health Organization.

Public-private partnerships Formal or informal joint endeavours involving state and non-state actors typically focused on a particular health policy issue or problem.

Quarantine The practice of isolating an individual who has or is suspected of having a disease, in order to prevent spreading the disease to others.

Regulation The enforcement of norms, standards, rules and principles which govern behaviour.

Regulatory capture The process by which an independent regulatory agency takes on the values and interests of the group whose activities it regulates.

Scenario A description of a set of conditions, either now, or, plausibly, in the future.

Smoking prevalence The percentage of a given population that currently smoke tobacco.

Sovereignty Supreme, exclusive power over the territory and people of a state.

Sustainable food supply A situation that ensures enough food of good quality, helps stimulate rural economies and promotes the social and environmental aspects of sustainable development.

Tariff A tax levied against an imported good or service.

Trade liberalization The process by which national economies become more open to cross-border flows of goods, services and capital.

Transnational corporation (TNC) A corporation that has developed coordinated control of its global business activities across national boundaries. This distinguishes the TNC from a multinational corporation (MNC), which operates in several countries but with limited coordination.

Transnational corporation A firm which owns branches in more than one country.

Vertical governance Governance that involves state and non-state actors above and below the sovereign state.

Weather Day-to-day climatic conditions versus longer-term conditions that define a prevailing *climate*.

Westphalian governance The framework for governing the relations among sovereign states that developed from the tenets of the Peace of Westphalia (1648).

Index

Page numbers in *italics* refer to figures and tables, those in **bold** indicate main discussion.